YOGA FOR NEW PARENTS

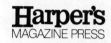

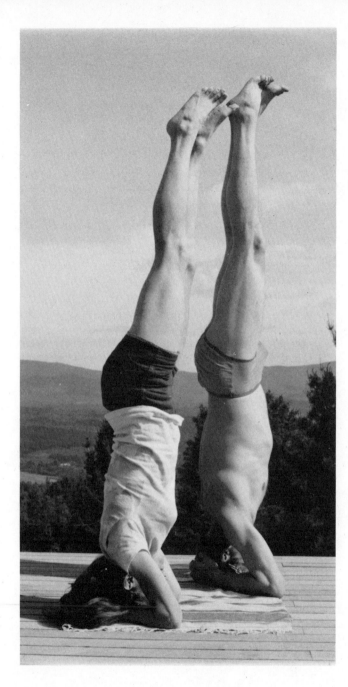

YOGA FOR NEW PARENTS

The Experience and the Practice

by Ferris Urbanowski, with Balaram

Charles W. Haney, photographer

HARPER'S MAGAZINE PRESS

Published in Association with Harper & Row

New York

Line drawings by Martim Avillez

Cover photographs by Rosemary Ranck and Charles W. Haney

YOGA FOR NEW PARENTS. Copyright © 1975 by Ferris B. Urbanowski. All rights reserved. Printed in the United States of America. No part of this book may be used or reproduced in any manner whatsoever without written permission except in the case of brief quotations embodied in critical articles and reviews. For information address Harper & Row, Publishers, Inc., 10 East 53rd Street, New York, N.Y. 10022. Published simultaneously in Canada by Fitzhenry & Whiteside Limited, Toronto.

FIRST EDITION

Cover and book design by C. Linda Dingler

Library of Congress Cataloging in Publication Data

Urbanowski, Ferris.
  Yoga for new parents.
  Bibliography: p.
  Includes index.
  1. Puerperium.　2. Muscle tone.　3. Yoga, Hatha.
I. Balaram, joint author.　II. Title.
RG801.U7　　613.7　　75-9355
ISBN 0-06-128300-2

75 76 77 78 79 10 9 8 7 6 5 4 3 2 1

To our students, who have taught us so much

CONTENTS

ABOUT THIS BOOK

When the extra ten pounds I had gained with my first baby stayed on after my second baby, I began to look for a way to lose weight (I'd never been very successful with dieting) and to regain some of the muscle tone I had lost during the two pregnancies.

I signed up for a yoga class. Though my first teacher did little more than present a few postures, I could see there was something to it. Then I moved from California to Pennsylvania, where I discovered the Center for Yogic Studies in Bucks County.

Under the tutelage of the director, Balaram, I lost ten pounds in a few months and the muscle tone of my newly flexible and relaxed body was vastly improved. I had more energy but was calmer; I felt less anxious and found myself enjoying and being more selective about each moment as I lived it.

I had experienced calmness and control, total involvement and joy, in my childbirth experiences. Now I began to see how yoga was directly related to the Lamaze preparation for childbirth, which I had used myself and had been teaching to others for six years. By practicing yoga, I began to have the same kind of control and awareness in my daily life.

Both yoga and the Lamaze method teach you to relax, to breathe, to focus.

Relaxation, so important in labor, ensures unrestricted circulation, slows the rate of breathing, and increases pain tolerance.

Breath control brings mastery of the body's energy and emotions. In the Lamaze method, various breathing patterns are used to cope with and control different parts of labor.

Focus centers the attention on total awareness of the now, alleviating anxieties and worries of past and future. In labor, the individual contraction can be dealt with; it is the worry about those to come—"Can I cope?"—that causes panic and loss of control.

The importance of these capabilities beyond the child-birth experience, and the teaching of them through yoga, was something I felt I must pass on. I talked with Balaram about a book that would similarly give others the opportunity to see the direct application of yoga to their daily lives.

As we talked and thought about the project, we discovered that there weren't any yoga books that applied to daily life situations.

Most books on yoga make it seem a unique, often esoteric, special thing, something to add to your life.

But the practice of yoga *is* life. The formal practice becomes one with daily life as the yogic states of relaxation, harmony of mind and body, calmness and concentration pervade one's entire being. When, through yoga practice, you begin to let go of all the tensions, anxieties, hopes, anticipations, and fears that bind you, you begin to have an awareness of the true Self—that part of you that is permanent and unchanging, that watches as you go through your daily actions, joys, disappointments, surprises, depressions. Awareness of that unchanging Self brings peace and places you in harmony with all life. Yoga does not add something to your life; rather, it reveals the true nature that was always there. Having this awareness doesn't make you perfect or change your personality. It does bring perspective, the ability to step back and look at yourself and your actions, to face difficulty and pain with equanimity.

People often think of yogis as recluses, living on remote mountaintops. To the contrary, the practice of yoga makes one able to do more to perform actions and to meet duties and responsibilities with greater effectiveness, concentration, and sureness.

What better time to begin yoga than during the advent of parenthood? Parenthood places one in new situations of stress, and imposes new obligations and responsibilities.

To reflect the total integration of day-to-day life and yoga, we decided to present the emotional aspects of pregnancy and parenthood, as well as actual yoga techniques. Though many of the emotions of this period are universal, each person has his or her own unique perspective on this important part of their lives. We decided our friends and students were the people to write this part of the book. We talked with a number of couples, during pregnancy and later, about their new roles as parents. The thoughts, actions, and emotions revealed in the "Pregnancy" and "Parenthood" sections are in their own words. It is their book. The yoga sections are our thanks and gift to them.

We would like to extend our deepest gratitude to all who gave so generously and openly of themselves to create this book. Particular thanks to Boz and Rusty Swope, who appear on both covers and throughout the book, and to their daughter, Rajah.

My own family, who appear in the "Regular Practice" section, have been very much a part of this project. When I first began yoga, my husband, Frank, watched for a while and then, seeing the results, began himself. Without my "Lamaze babies," Alexandra, now 11, and Tasha, 9, none of it would have ever happened.

The patience and persistence of our photographer, Chuck Haney, and his wife, Abby, made a project that could have been tedious and difficult a happening of pleasure and camaraderie.

My goddaughter, Trilby MacDonald, is responsible for the book's publication. It was at her baby shower that I met Gwyneth Cravens of *Harper's Magazine*, who saw the book's potential, took the idea to Harper's Magazine Press, and, with talent and grace, midwifed it into being.

The candid sections of the book, "Pregnancy" and "Parenthood," are meant to be experienced as you wish.

The four yoga sections are to be done sequentially.

The woman begins a few simple, effective postures the first day after giving birth. After the first week, she and her husband are ready to start with "Beginning at Home."

Movement from "Beginning at Home" to "When You Have It Going" should be at the individual's own pace. When all the postures in one section can be easily accomplished, you are ready to move to the next. You will notice that many of the postures in one section are repeated in the next, simpler postures are replaced by slightly more difficult ones, and new ones are added. Each section is built on the one preceding until the "Regular Practice" section, which gives an ongoing practice routine. (We do not represent this routine as a fully developed Hatha Yoga program. Consult the bibliography for further information.) The index provides a quick reference to the routine of each section.

You may spend several weeks or months in each section. Do not push yourself! Go at your own pace, but be consistent in your practice.

If you want to share the book with older parents, or with nonparents, people of any age, "When You Have It Going" is a good place to begin. Be sure they read "The Practice" section first.

Peace   Om Shanthi

FERRIS URBANOWSKI

Buckeye Knoll, 1975

EXPERIENCE

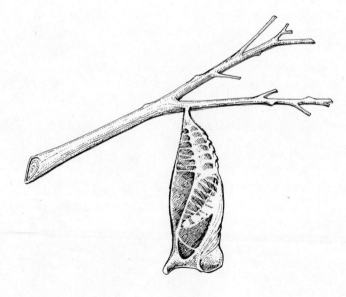

PREGNANCY

The birth of a child is one of life's most important transitional events for mother, father, and child. The child may forget, but for mother and father the character and quality of the experience are of major importance.

A woman must form a view of herself as a mother, as a caretaker. Her independence is gone for years to come, lost in the responsibilities of motherhood and child care. She must reach out beyond herself, beyond her relationship to the child's father, to give love—unqualified love—to yet another being, a being whose very existence is dependent on her.

The pregnancy itself is a constant reminder that the transformation from woman to mother is taking place. The changes in her body—tender breasts, a full feeling in the abdomen, nausea, fatigue, frequency of urination—make her aware of an altered state of being before her mate has begun to realize or accept the pregnancy. He can only listen, observe, reflect. He can't feel what's happening within her. He may start to worry about the new responsibilities a child will bring, about money, about changes in his life, but it is all not quite real, not immediate.

Initially, both man and woman experience ambivalence about the pregnancy, whether it was planned or unplanned. Their lives, individually and together, begin to shift and change as the experience of pregnancy and the anticipation of parenthood deepen. The awareness of a changed and changing state of being is unsettling to the most stable of individuals and marriages. Its effect on the less stable can be irrevocable.

With the advent of the baby as a personality, in the form of a bulging abdomen, flutters, movements, and finally kicks, the pregnancy becomes a reality for both mother and father.

For the woman, the second three months of pregnancy usually bring a physical and mental high—a minute-to-minute sense of being more than oneself: she is

4

truly united with another being. Only the sexual act—at its most complete—approaches the unity of being experienced in pregnancy.

Spiritual seekers spend years training their bodies and minds as they search for enlightenment, satori, samadhi—a total oneness, perfect balance, complete unity. Pregnancy can offer a glimpse of what these states might be.

With pregnancy an unalterable reality, the man becomes more aware, and more involved. As his wife feels increasingly vulnerable and dependent, both physically and emotionally, he may feel trapped and frightened. He may also respond to the joy of new life, to the woman who is more than herself, to the bonding of the two of them through a state of being that is of, yet more than, both of them.

Often the couple experiences heightened sexuality and, in the sexual act, amusement at the physical obstacles, lack of fear of becoming pregnant, a feeling that there's someone else there with them, a freewheeling joy in knowing that the pregnancy has made something between them more complete.

During the last three months, as pregnancy nears its completion and climax—birth—anxiety and anticipation about the rite of passage, the birth itself, are mixed with pride and fulfillment in the state of being "great with child." Many women feel beatific and transcendent during the latter part of pregnancy.

As the approaching event becomes the substance of their daily lives, the man becomes an intrinsic part of the happening. Although he cannot share the woman's physical experience, and may still have anxious moments of feeling trapped and burdened, he usually gets caught up in the excitement and anticipation. Preparations are accelerated. If the couple is attending preparation for childbirth classes, his involvement becomes more active and meaningful for both of them. Through the classes, he learns about the labor and delivery process, the woman's feelings and experience, and how to play an active and useful role in the birth of his child. As the couple practices and prepares together, a special intimacy envelops them.

As individuals, and together, they approach birth; the rite of passage for both of them from independent male to father, from independent female to mother, from lovers to parents.

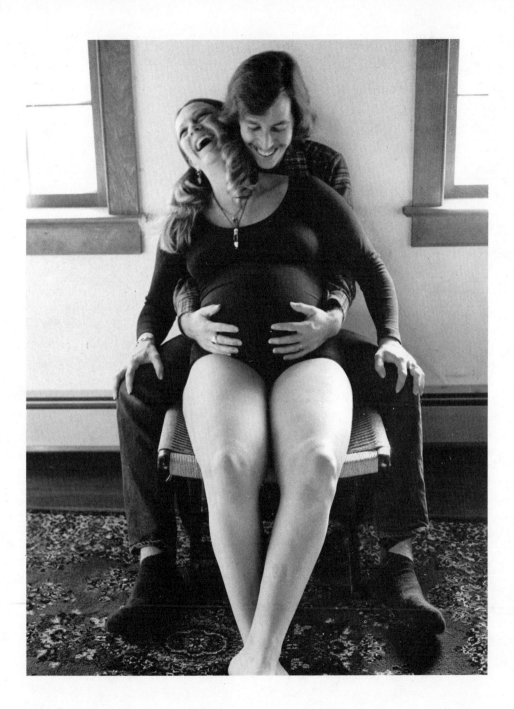

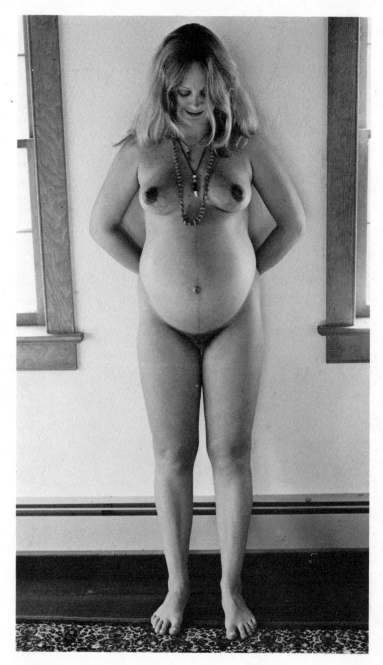

I'm amazed my body can get so big! When I was six months along, I couldn't believe I could get any bigger!

Sex is a whole new trip. It's something else to be kicked from inside while you're making love.

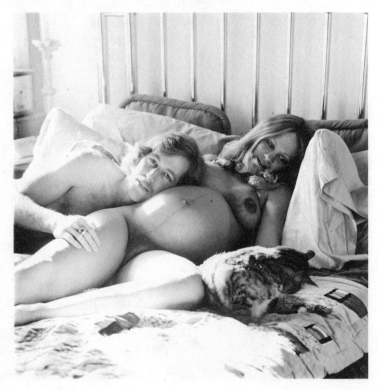

8

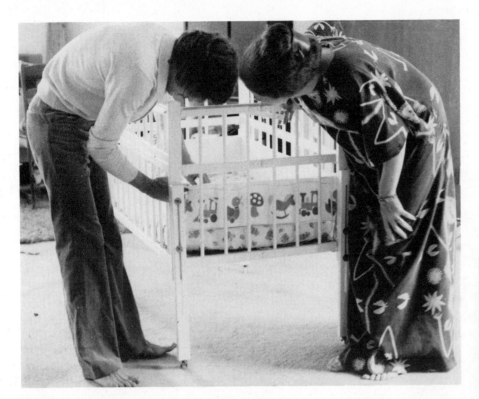

It still doesn't seem quite real. I'm as big as a house, it jumps around all day, and our room is beginning to fill with baby things. But I still can't believe there's going to be a baby.

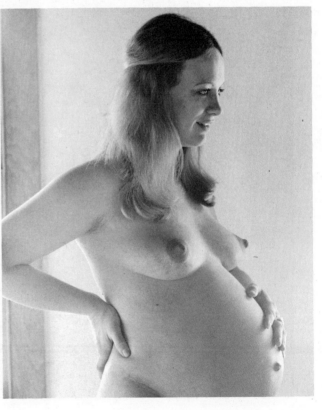

In a dream I saw its face, its eyes. It was a girl, laughing and happy. I carried her around with me everywhere. I had a real sense of her as a person. When I woke up, I felt so happy.

At first I had a strong sensation of fear. There's so much responsibility. But I realized that was selfishness, a fear of extending myself.

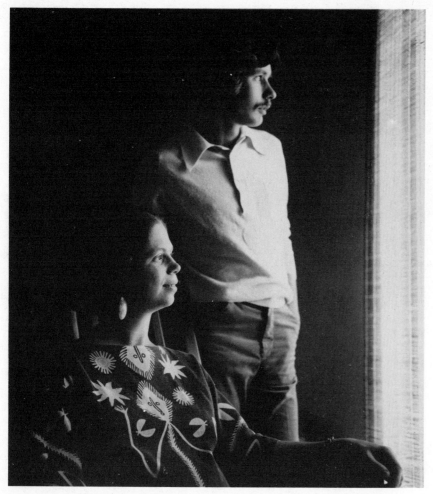

Almost all societies recognize the importance of the father's involvement in the birth of his child.

Some societies even give him vicarious physical participation—called couvade—which transfers the maternal aspects of birth to the father. Among the Bantu of Africa, for instance, the husband takes to his bed and is tended by his wife for a week following the birth of their baby.

In our society, most men are impressed with and sometimes nearly overwhelmed by a sense of tremendous responsibility: responsibility for the child, economically and as a father figure, and responsibility toward their mate.

Being on the outside is often harder: the man must work to imagine what it's like to be pregnant and to give birth, while the woman feels it all, knows it all.

At a time when the man may feel very insecure, his mate is highly dependent on him. Yet, despite the demands and stress, pregnancy can be a time of special intimacy.

I used to be very insecure about going places alone. Now that I've become more than myself, I feel invulnerable and beautiful. I feel I could go anywhere and do anything.

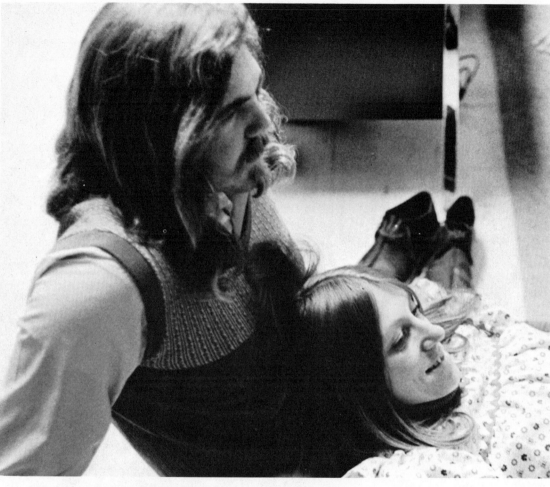

*My wife . . . now she's two of her. She's carrying our child
and I feel terrible. I want to help her, but there's nothing I
can do for her. That's the strongest emotion I've felt
throughout . . .* HELPLESSNESS!

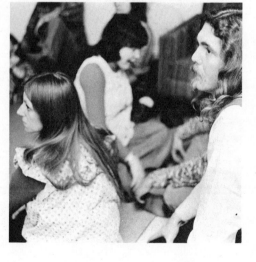

*I'm not sure I'm ready for this at all; sometimes I feel so
trapped.*

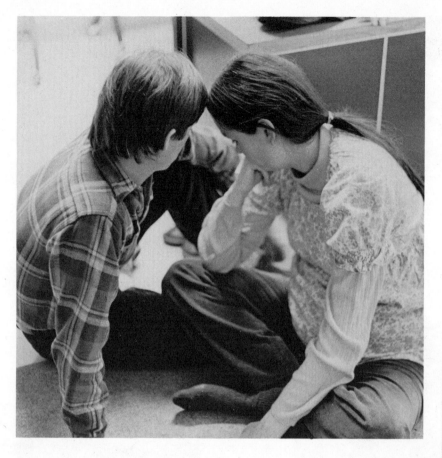

We've tried to imagine what the combination of the two of us would be like. . . .

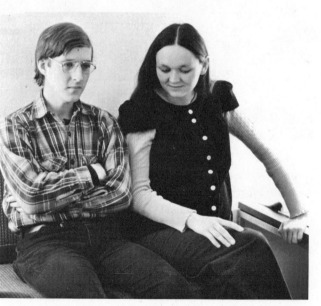

There's a great joy in the consciousness of helping a human being to evolve. I look forward to that responsibility.

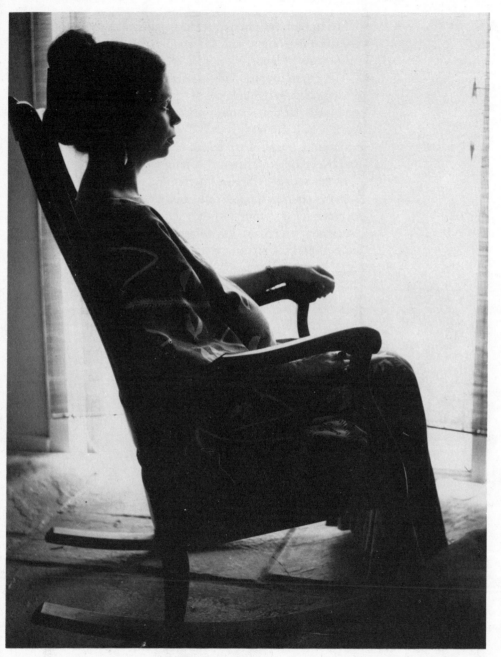

At the beginning I was always aware of being pregnant, now I'm always aware that I'm going into labor. What will it be like, will I get through it . . . ?

13

Preparation for childbirth classes do much more than prepare the woman, and the couple, for the physiological process of labor.

The group support and sharing that is so much a part of these classes reminds me of the tribe where the entire extended family—aunts, uncles, cousins—arrives a week before the birth is due. Tents are set up, elaborate community meals are cooked, children play, dogs bark, and everybody catches up on family news.

In our society, where a functioning extended family is a rarity, couples support one another, sometimes in the intimacy of a community life style, more often in the artificially structured environment of a class. But the support and the sharing are there!

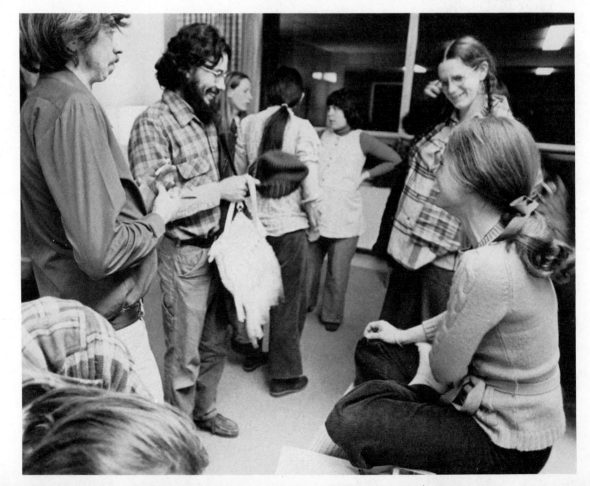

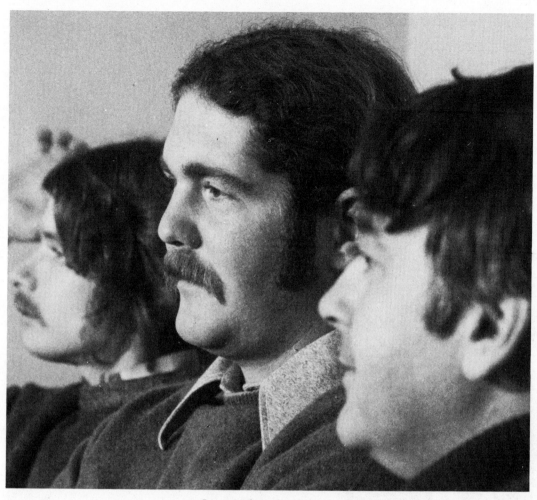

I never thought the man could be anything but useless during the birth itself. When she said she wanted to take these classes, and I had to come along too, I was very hesitant. To see other men there, and hear they were dragged along too, was reassuring.
I'm finding out there's a lot I can learn about birth and about helping her. I'm beginning to feel I can be a real help during the labor.

The body is relaxed, and the arm swings back and forth without any resistance. The mind is focused on watching the breath as it flows in and out.

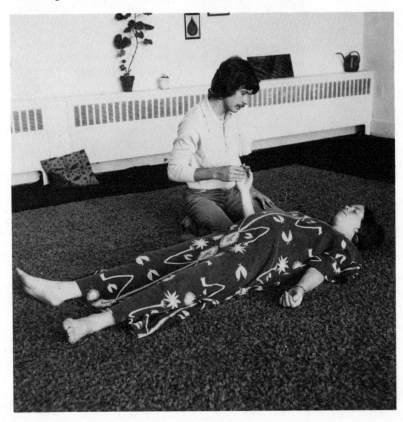

Relax . . . focus . . . breathe. These three concepts are essential for preparing for labor—and for dealing with life.

The body is naturally relaxed and calm—it is tension in the mind that makes tension and rigidity in the body.

By freeing the mind of fears and misconceptions, and by learning to consciously relax, the woman can approach labor with a body whose relaxed state allows the process of labor—hundreds of minute-long contractions of the uterus that open the neck of the womb, widen the cervix, and finally push the baby into the outside world—to occur with maximum efficiency.

By focusing her attention on dealing with each individual contraction rather than on future contractions, she can become one with it, accepting it, riding with it as a surfer rides the wave.

Her support is her breathing. Every emotional state has a corresponding rate of respiration. By breathing in particular ways during the various stages and phases of labor, she regulates her emotions, staying calm and controlled, letting go so the labor can progress. Her regulated breathing ensures that the baby is receiving adequate oxygen and helps her to adjust to the increasing intensity of the contractions as the labor approaches its climax.

When the baby is ready to be born, the mother controls her breath and, in an orchestrated motion of the diaphragm, abdominal muscles, and vagina, pushes the baby out through the birth canal.

To learn about her body, the feeling of tension as opposed to relaxation, and to simulate the contracted state of the uterus during labor, the woman contracts a selected muscle or muscle group while her partner—who will be her coach in labor—checks to make sure that the rest of her body is completely relaxed.

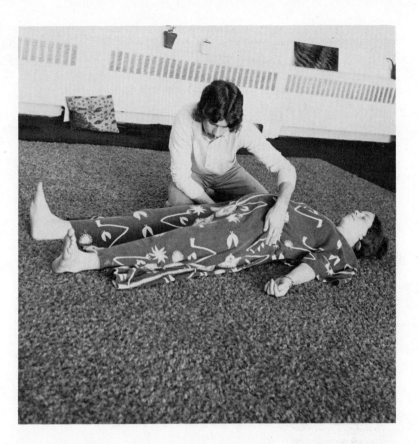

"Contract both legs." Be sure the lower back is relaxed. The baby presses against the lower back during labor, making it hard to keep it relaxed.

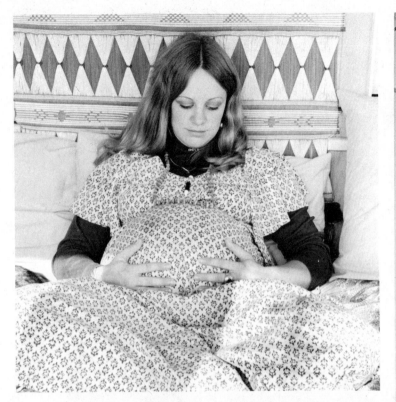

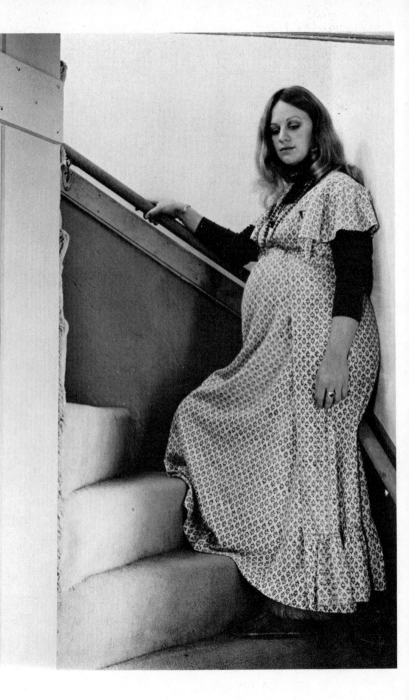

I had a wonderful dream that the baby's foot came out through my stomach, a perfectly formed foot and leg, and I played with it, and felt so happy. It seemed so right.

Everything is so sore! My ribs feel bruised and battered. Everything on the bottom feels delicate and swollen. Every once in a while I get these shooting pains inside, as if the baby is jumping on top of my cervix.

Sleeping is a problem too. I just can't seem to get comfortable, and then, of course, there are the trips to the bathroom. Being tired makes it hard for me to control my emotions. I feel right at the edge.

18

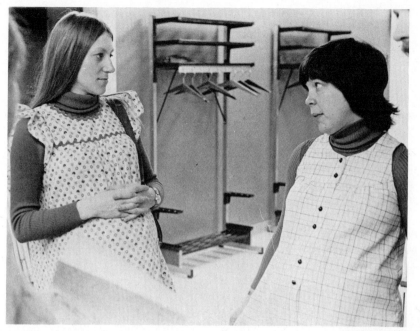

Every once in a while I panic about the labor. I guess there's no way out but through it. I look at the other people in my class, and I figure if they can do it, I can. And I suppose I will.

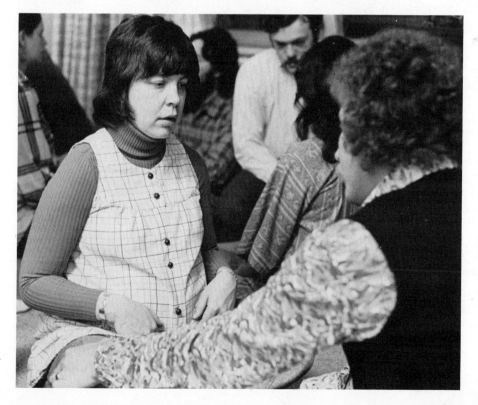

The classes are helping. I know I'm doing my best to prepare. I'll know what's happening, and if this stuff works the way it's supposed to, I'll know what to do.

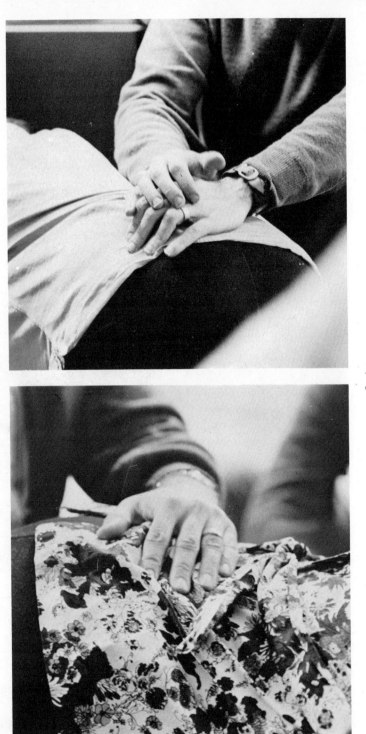

I hope it's not back labor! I don't know how long either one of us could keep it up.

20

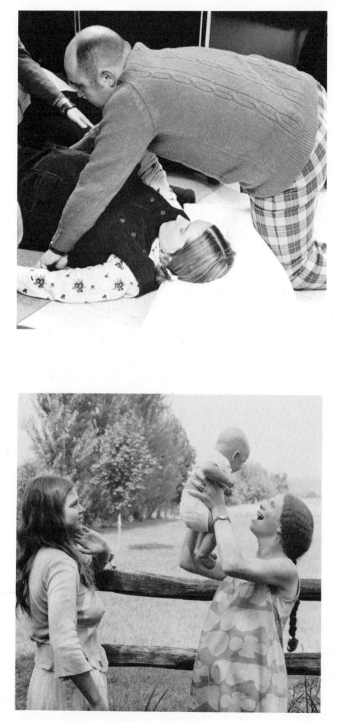

I feel confident that I'll know what to do. Knowing what's happening helps. You should have heard me telling my mother all about the stages and phases of labor.

I have the feeling I can't go anywhere. The other day I was walking to the movies and I suddenly realized: "Hey, you can't just disappear for a few hours at a time. It could be any minute!"

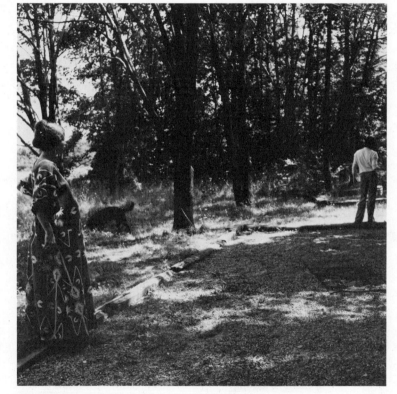

The waiting is driving me nuts! I have this image of his just having driven off to work—an hour away—and me running after him yelling, "Stop, wait, I'm in labor!"

I felt really confident until about a week ago, but now that I know it can be any time, I'm not so sure. I keep looking at other women and babies and thinking, well, they lived through it. . . .

21

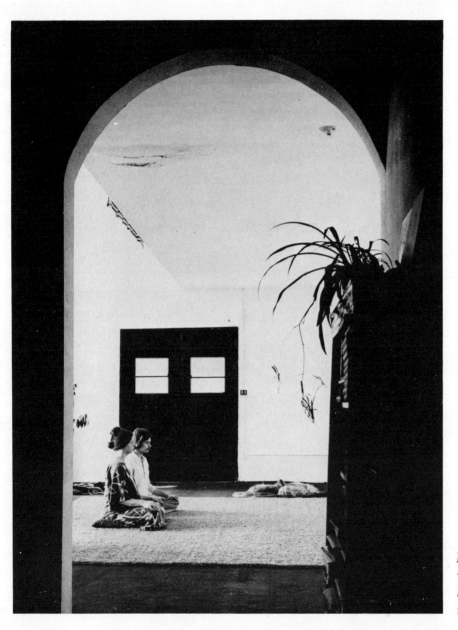

It feels like being suspended. You know what you're waiting for, but you don't know exactly what it will be like, how it will start, where you'll be, how you'll react. . . .

BIRTH

All births are the same and all births
are different.
All births are holy. We thank you,
O Lord, this gift of life.

—*Eugene*
Two Births

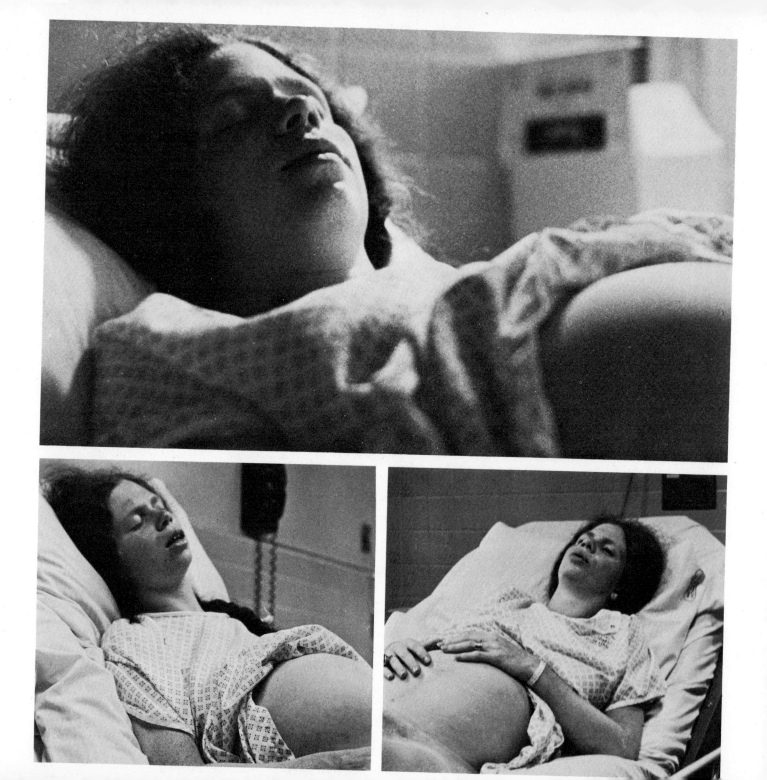

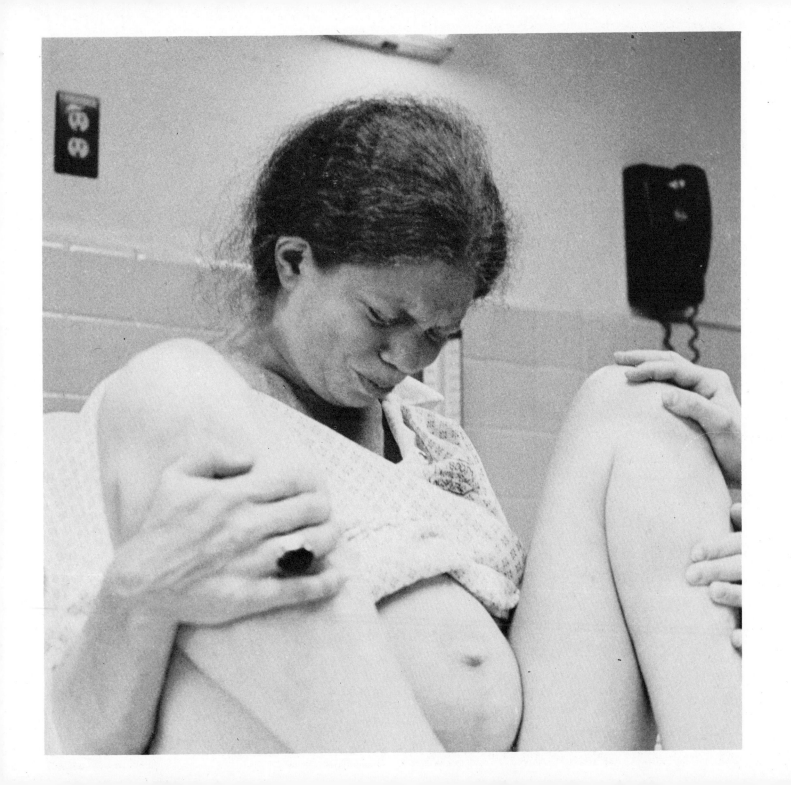

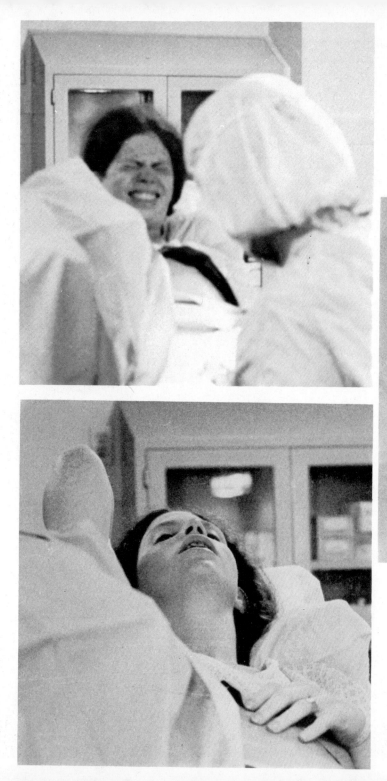
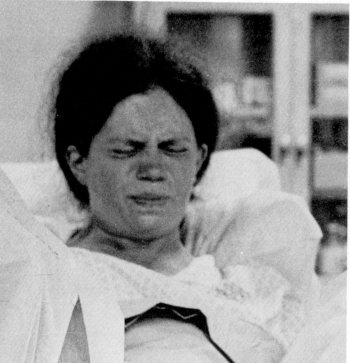

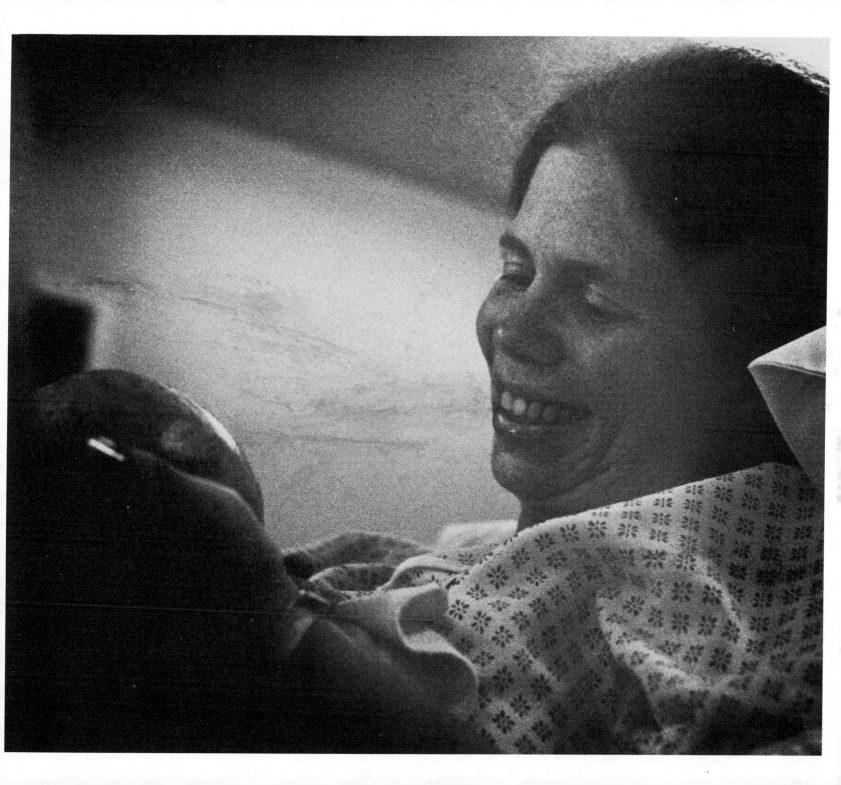

PRACTICE

By letting go, it all gets done.
The world is won by those who let it go.
But when you try and try, it is ever beyond
the winning.

—Tao te Ching

HOW TO START

The origins of yoga are not really known. The first written evidence of the yogic disciplines is contained in India's scriptures, some of which are more than six thousand years old. We know that an oral tradition existed for the purpose of passing on the knowledge from teacher to student for centuries before any of it was put into writing.

Basically, there are five major yogas, each concerning itself with developing an aspect of personality. Hatha Yoga, the yoga of physical perfection, brings control of the body and its energy; Raja Yoga is the yoga of meditation and mind control, which is distinguished from Jnana Yoga, or the yoga of the intellect. Bhakti Yoga develops the emotions as an aspect of meditation—it is easy to concentrate on something or someone we love. Karma Yoga is the yoga of action, helping us to perform action with equanimity and nonattachment.

Here we are concerned mainly with Hatha Yoga and a little Raja Yoga, as an introduction to meditation. The divisions between one type of yoga and another are really to make talking about it easier. Actually they are not separate systems. There is always a mixture of several or all of the yogas in each discipline. For example, Hatha Yoga appears to be just a physical discipline, but Raja Yoga is also present, as it takes concentration of the mind (Raja Yoga) to do the postures correctly.

The goal of all the yogic systems, whether through the intellect, mind, body control, or through the emotions, is to realize the true Self. This state of realization is the same no matter how it is reached.

"Truth is One. Paths are many," said Swami Satchidananda.

Self is One.
There is only one Self—one consciousness.
It only appears to be divided.
We can have many ideas about the Self, but the idea
  is never It.

The Self is not an idea.
Self is something very definite.
Self is not body.
Self is not mind.
Self is not ego.
Self is not emotion.
Self is not the thought "I."
Self is the part of your personality that always remains
  the same.

"There's nothing about me that stays the same," you
may say. "My mind changes, my body changes, my
feelings change."
  But who is aware of change?
  What is this awareness?
  This awareness *is* Self!
  So, even though the mind changes, the body changes,
the awareness of it all is constant, that is Self—you.
  The goal of yoga is realization of the Self, or the
original nature, or true Self.
  The true Self is peaceful, complete, and happy.
  If each of us has a true Self, why don't we feel this
peace? Because of anxiety, stress, attachment; in other
words, not letting go . . . getting caught in the tension,
in the worry . . .

  The event of childbirth places stress on every aspect of
the new parents' personalities: physical (especially for the
laboring mother), mental, and emotional. Knowledge
that this event has just begun and realization of the
sacrifices and responsibilities involved can create more
strain than many parents feel they can handle.
  The physical discomforts of tension and stiffness are
caused by the stressed mind, which transfers its anxiety
to the body. However, this nervous energy in the body
can be controlled. You can stop its flow to the muscles.
The yogic disciplines offer release from and control over
physical, mental, and emotional strains. Yoga postures

help your body unlearn rigidity and tension so that your natural calm emerges.

Calmness brings the ability to focus on the actions of the here and now, on this moment. This is the real and only meaning of meditation.

All the yogic techniques help you to let go . . . to practice them *is* to let go. It's not so easy to be relaxed. Habitually, unconsciously, we tend to tense first this part of the body, then that part. In letting go you actually gain control over yourself in a wider sense.

Savasana . . . the corpse pose . . . just like a corpse, the body is completely limp. . . .

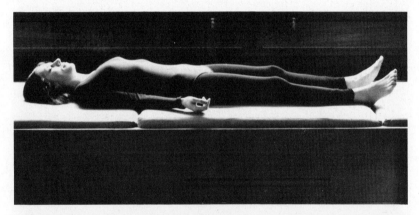

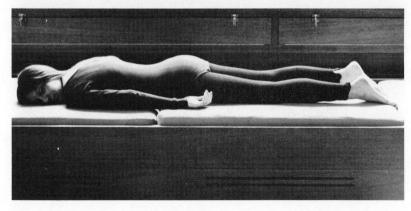

The Corpse Pose (Savasana)

Let the body go . . .
Just allow everything to relax.
Separate the feet . . . relax the legs . . .
Have the palms turned up, arms limp . . .
Close the eyes . . .
Focus the attention within . . .
Let go . . . even of the breath . . .
Let the breath flow by itself . . .
Just watch the breath flow in and out . . .

Savasana is done between most of the asanas.

Every Savasana should be a complete relaxation, but only for thirty seconds to a minute. Don't fall asleep!

Each time you return to Savasana . . . relax!

Let go . . . stop tensing . . . even the smallest muscles are relaxed. . . .

Focus within . . . watch the breath.

THREE-PART BREATHING

There should be one smooth movement filling up the entire trunk from the belly to the chest, emptying from the chest to the belly.

Inhale *slowly,*

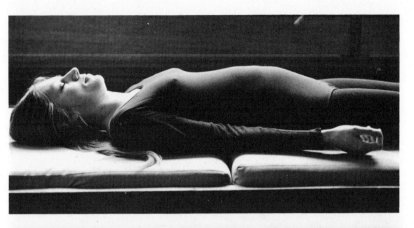

Expand just the belly . . . push it all the way out . . .

Continue . . . expand the ribs, filling the middle chest . . .

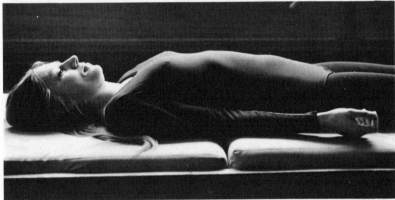

Now inhale all the way . . . push out the chest, even raising the collarbones.

Exhale *slowly,*

Drop the collarbones . . .
Pull in the ribs, empty the middle chest . . .
Pull in the belly, forcing out all the air . . .

And again . . .
Inhale *slowly,*
expand the belly . . . ribs . . . chest . . .
Exhale *slowly,*
chest . . . ribs . . . belly.

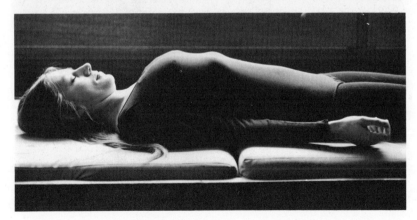

Three-part breathing means using your entire body to breathe. This is difficult for most people. Constriction in the abdomen keeps them from using their entire lung capacity.

Three-part breathing oxygenates the blood, allowing the rate of respiration and pulse to slow down.

It is the preparation for pranayama (energy control). It teaches control of the movement of the breath from the belly.

Pranayama centers the body's vital forces.

MEDITATIVE POSES

The purpose of the meditative pose is to give a firm and comfortable seat. This enables one to temporarily forget the body and concentrate within.

Finding this firm, comfortable seat is difficut, if not impossible in the beginning!

Practice in sitting, plus Hatha Yoga, will bring the physical mastery that makes meditation possible.

Some meditative poses, starting with the easier ones, follow.

The Comfortable Pose (Sukhasana)

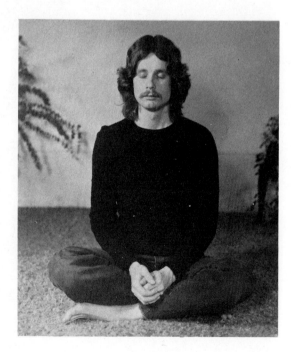

Sit on the floor with the legs stretched forward (you may sit on a cushion),

Comfortably cross the legs under the thighs,

Fold the hands in the lap,

Keep the head, neck, trunk in a straight line. Try to keep the spine vertical without tensing the legs . . .

Eyes closed. . . .

The Pelvic Pose (Vajrasana)

   Kneel on the floor, keeping the knees together,
   Sit down on the feet with the toes touching and the heels
apart . . .
   Hands on the knees or folded in the lap,
   Back straight . . .
   Eyes closed. . . .

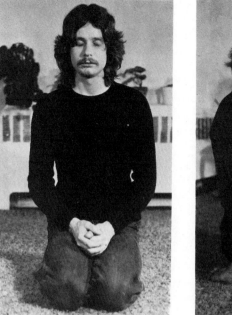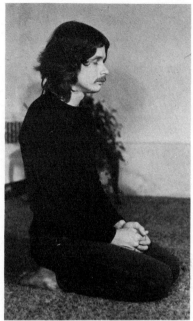

The Half-Lotus (Arddha Padmasana)

   Sit on the floor with the legs stretched forward,
   Place one foot on top of the thigh, pull the foot as close
to the abdomen as you can,
   Bring the other foot underneath the thigh,
   Hands on the knees or folded in the lap,
   Back straight . . .
   Eyes closed. . . .

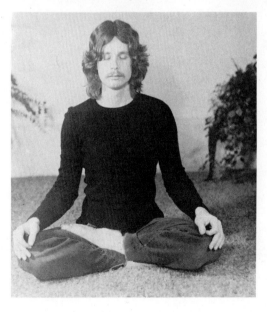

The Lotus Pose (Padmasana)

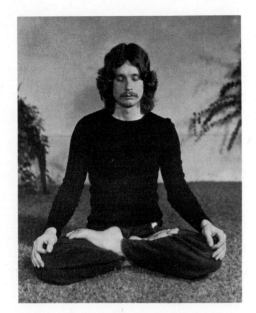

Sit on the floor with the legs stretched forward,
Place one foot on top of the thigh, pull the foot as close
to the abdomen as you can,
Bring the other foot on top of the thigh,
Hands on the knees or folded in the lap . . .
Back straight . . .
Eyes closed. . . .

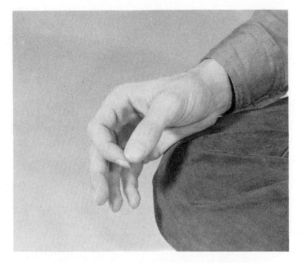

THE MUDRAS

Mudra is a Sanskrit word meaning "seal."
The hand mudras are refinements in the asana (meditation posture) which help focus the vital force (prana) and aid the mind in arriving at concentration.

Chin Mudra

The heel of the hand rests on the knee.
Join the index finger and thumb, gently letting them touch.
The other fingers are relaxed.

Chin Mudra (Variation)

Tuck the index finger into the base of the thumb. . . .

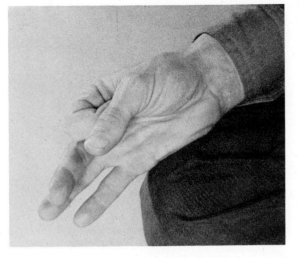

Yoga Mudra

(Do before and after meditation)
Put the hands behind the back, have a grasp on one
wrist,
Straighten the spine,
Close the eyes,
Exhale and fold all the way forward,
Keep the seat firmly on the floor
(Hold 30 seconds to a minute) . . .
Let the head drop, shoulders relaxed . . .
and
Slowly raise the head,
Sit up,
Open the eyes. . . .

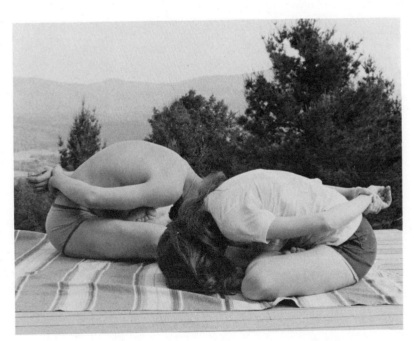

AFTER THE BIRTH

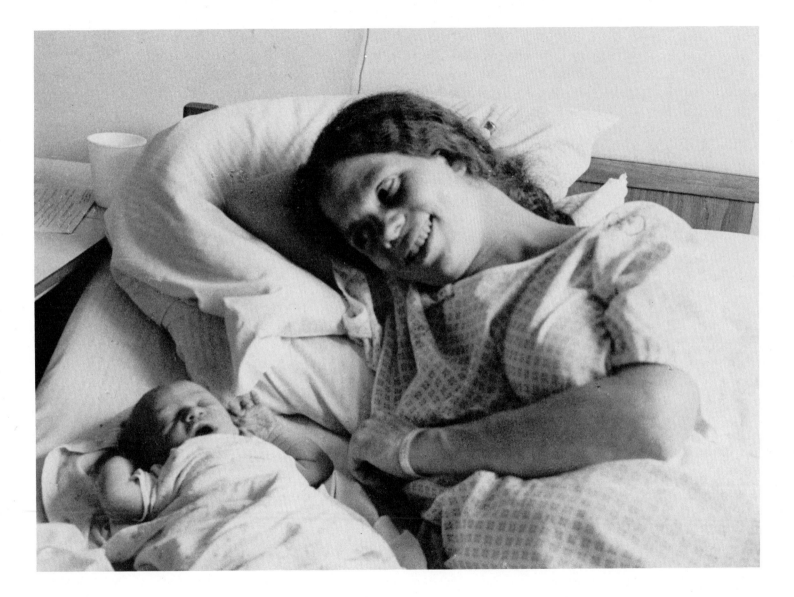

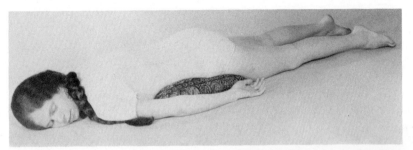

Start Practicing *Now*, While You're Still in The Hospital

Now is the time to begin.

While your daily needs are being taken care of, take some time to focus on yourself.

Evaluate:

No longer pregnant,

But certainly not returned to a familiar body.

An empty, flabby belly

(the muscle tone will, with a little effort, come back),

Soreness!

Bruised bottom,

Full, sensitive breasts,

Bloody flow, even clots of surprising size.

Begin now to make a time each day, just for yourself.

You'll need it in the busy weeks and months to come.

Start working with your body,

Begin to know it anew.

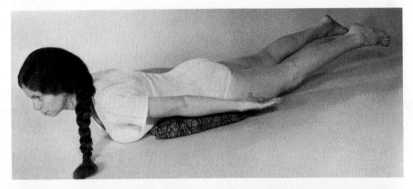

Savasana on the Stomach

Put a pillow under the belly to prevent pressure on the breasts.

Relax in this position frequently during the first few days after giving birth.

Back Stretch

Stretch from head to toe, tensing all the muscles of the back.

Repeat four times, resting in Savasana between each stretch.

Savasana on the back.

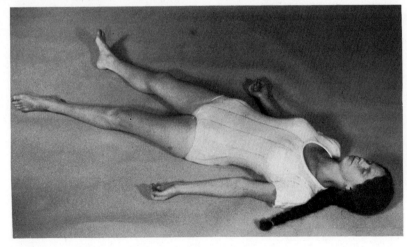

Take a Few Three-Part Breaths

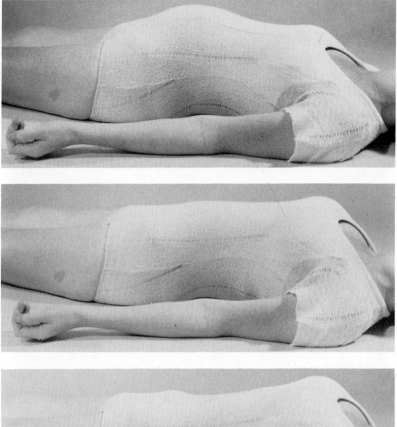

Pelvic Floor Contractions

While lying in Savasana, contract the vagina slowly, firmly, and with increasing intensity, as if you were going up in an elevator.

Begin tightening: 1—2—3—4—5—tightly contracted . . .

Now release slowly and with control: 5—4—3—2—1.

Repeat twenty times daily.

If you have trouble identifying the proper muscles, try when you are urinating to stop the flow in midstream. The muscles you contract to do that are the right ones.

Because of the stretching of these muscles during birth, it may be hard to feel them working for a few days. Keep at it!

The more you do this exercise, the more rapidly these important muscles will regain tone and strength. If you've had stitches, doing this exercise will help the healing process.

For good muscle tone and increased sexual response, do this exercise twenty times daily for the rest of your life!

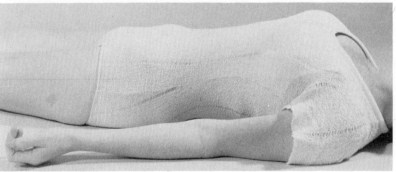

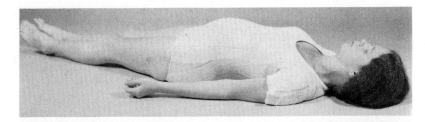

Head Lift

Slowly inhale through the nose, pushing out the belly.

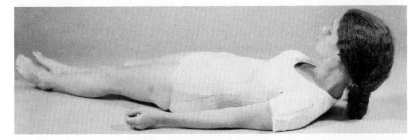

Raise the head, exhaling through the lips.
Draw the belly in and down as hard as possible.
Repeat.
Return to Savasana . . . feet apart, palms turned up . . . relax. . . .

Pelvic Rock

Bend the knees, feet flat on the bed.
Take a relaxed inhalation,
Exhale, pressing back and shoulders firmly against the bed, pull in the belly as tightly as possible.

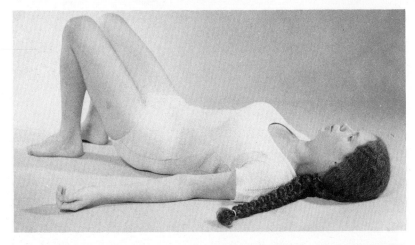

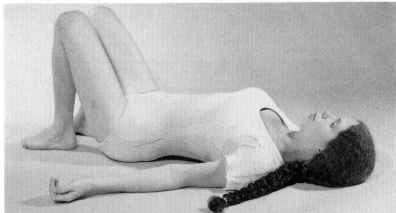

Inhale, relaxing abdomen, back, and shoulders.
Repeat three times on the first day after delivery; add one more pelvic rock daily until the sixth day.
Continue to do this exercise six times daily for at least a month.
Extend the legs . . .
Savasana. . . .

Quick Relaxation

Note: Try reading the instructions several times to get an idea of the method and flow in relaxation, then start practicing by reading it aloud to each other.

Savasana . . . let the body go. . . .

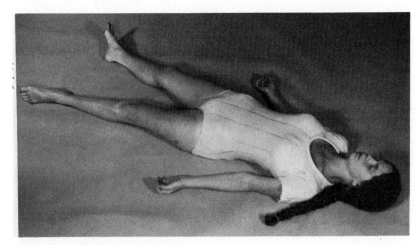

Keep the feet apart, arms at the sides, and,
Stretch out! Stretch the legs and arms, push the feet away from the body, push the hands away. . . .

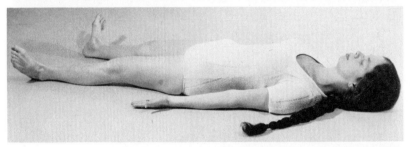

Inhale! Hold the breath, make fists, tense the whole body—arms, legs, chest, shoulders . . .
Raise the arms, legs, and head . . .
Full tension!
Exhale through a wide open mouth,
Drop to the floor . . . relax. . . .

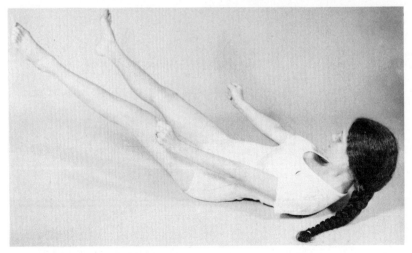

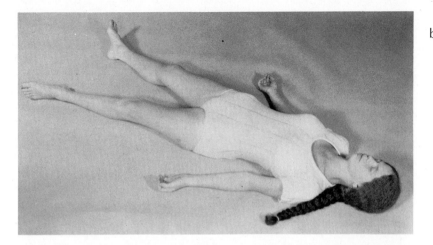

Tense the muscles of the buttocks, almost raising the body off the floor . . . relax. . . .

Inhale! Push the abdomen all the way out, trap the air in the belly . . .
Exhale, mouth wide open . . . relax. . . .

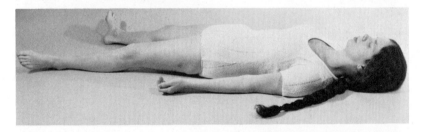

Inhale again, push out the chest . . .
Exhale . . . relax. . . .

Push the shoulders up toward the chin
(not the ears!) . . .
Relax. . . .

Push the face up; imagine you are pushing the muscles of the face toward the nose . . .
Relax. . . .

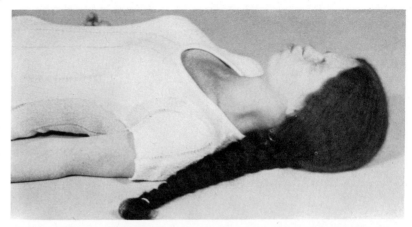

Stretch the face, open the eyes, mouth wide open, push the tongue out as far as it will go. . . .
Relax.

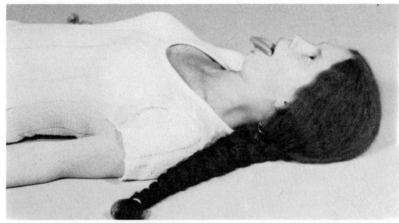

Make any adjustments in the position now so you can *completely* let the body go.

From this point on, make a strong resolve not to move the body until Quick Relaxation is over.

Starting with the feet . . . keep your attention on them, feeling that you've let them go completely, not moving even the smallest muscles.

Now the ankles and calves . . . let them go . . .

Bring your attention to the knees and thighs . . . knees and thighs completely relaxed . . .

The entire legs, ankles, and feet are let go.

Now the hands . . . hands and wrists relaxed . . .
Then the forearms . . . then the upper arms . . .
The entire arms, wrists, hands, relaxed.

Go from the limbs to the trunk.

First, the lower trunk relaxes . . . feel as if the weight of the lower trunk just sinks into the floor . . .

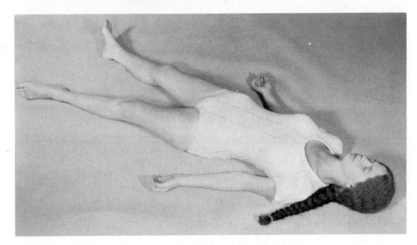

Now the middle trunk . . . let the middle back and abdomen relax . . .

Then up to the chest and upper back . . . everything let go . . . relax . . . completely limp.

From the trunk go up to the shoulders . . . shoulders relaxed . . .

Now the neck, and finally the face . . . let all the muscles of the face go slack . . . face relaxed.

Keep your attention within the body, watch the breath . . . let it flow in . . . let it flow out . . . don't control it . . . just watch . . .

Every time the mind wanders, bring it back to the breath.

(3 to 5 minutes)

Inhale and exhale deeply about ten times,

Roll the arms and legs back and forth,

Roll the head back and forth, waking the body up,

Slowly sit up.

BEGINNING AT HOME

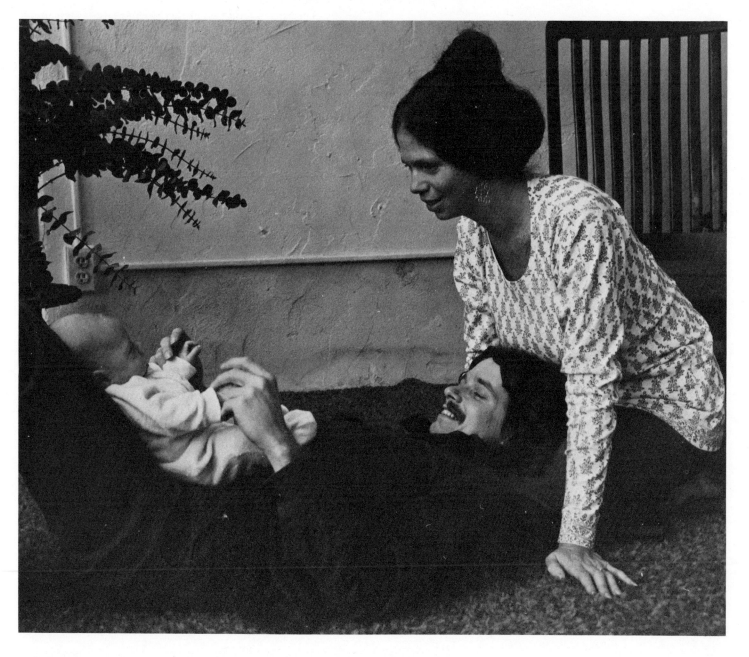

Don't wait!

Do it *now!*

A child is an ongoing, ever-present part of your life.

Parenthood has become your state of being.

Deal with it now, don't let it overwhelm you.

Make time for yourself each day.

Practice while the baby sleeps, or have someone else look after him, or just let the baby *be* for an hour—he doesn't need to be watched or cared for every minute.

If you don't do it now, it will get harder and harder.

You'll find yourself without privacy, and with less and less patience.

By making time for reflection, calmness, you will grow as a person and as a parent.

The best time is early morning. You may be stiff—don't be discouraged. You'll notice that our models are not always doing the poses perfectly.

You haven't eaten (yoga should not be done after eating).

You set your mood for the whole day.

In these first few weeks, when the baby has no schedule, do it when you can, but *do* it!

Perhaps you and your husband—or a friend—can read the instructions to each other. It's a good way to begin to get the flow of the practice.

Make sure the room is well ventilated, and wear comfortable, easy-to-move-in clothing.

Focus your attention as you do each posture,

Never strain, never push, let your body relax into the pose.

While in the posture, run over your body with the mind, relaxing tense muscles,

Concentrate.

Enjoy the practice.

Begin with Savasana on the back,

Relax . . .

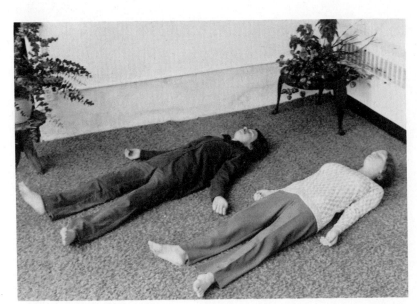

Let the entire weight settle into the floor.
Take a few minutes to let the whole body relax. . . .
(2 to 3 minutes)

Start with three-part breathing . . .
Remember! Inhale from the belly first,
Exhale from the belly last. . . .
(5 minutes)

Turn over,
Savasana on the stomach . . .
Relax. . . .

Half-Locust (Arddha Salabasana)

Bring the arms underneath the body, thighs resting on the upturned palms, elbows close together under the trunk.
Lift the right leg, keeping it straight.
Hold 30 seconds to a minute, slowly lower the leg, and . . .
Repeat with the left leg . . .
Bring the arms out from under the body . . .
Savasana . . . feet apart . . . palms turned up.

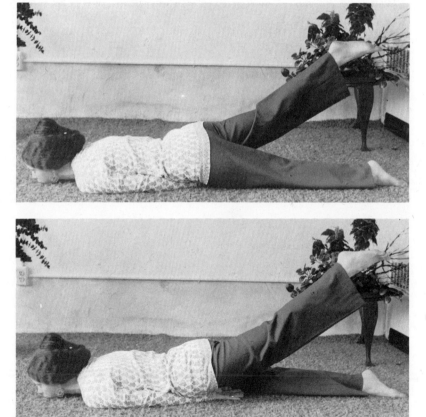

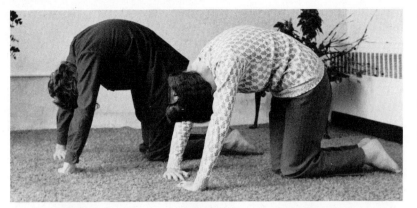

Cat and Cow Pose

The Cat and Cow Pose is really closer to an exercise than an asana.

The spine is flexed from a fully arched (the cat) to a swayback pose (the cow).

Stand on the hands and knees, fingers pointing inward . . .

Drop the head, exhaling forcefully through the nose.

Push the back all the way up (toward the ceiling). . . .

Inhale! Pull the head back,

Drop the spine (toward the floor),

and

Exhale, drop the head, push the back up,

Inhale, pull the head back, drop the spine. . . .

Repeat ten times.

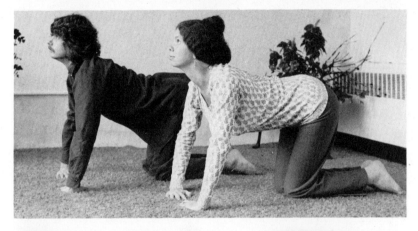

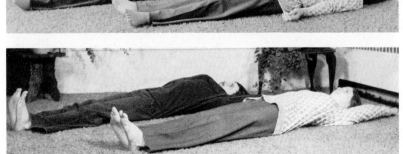

Savasana on the back. . . .

Full Forward Bending (Paschimothanasana)

Savasana on the back. . . .

Bring the feet together,

Stretch the arms over the head (on the floor),

Lock thumbs, stretch. . . .

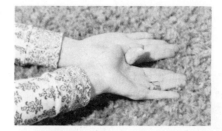

Sit up (using the elbows for support if necessary), stretch for the ceiling,
    Inhale,
    and

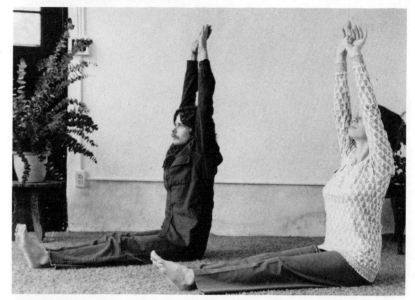

Exhale, drop all the way forward,
    Grasp the legs (keep the arms bent), drop the head, drop the shoulders,
    Relax into the asana with every exhalation.
    (Hold for 1 minute)
    Lock thumbs, reach for the feet, stretch for the ceiling,
    Stretch . . .
    and
    arms at the sides . . .

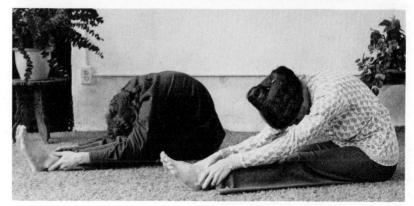

Head-to-Knee Pose (Janu-Sirs Asana)

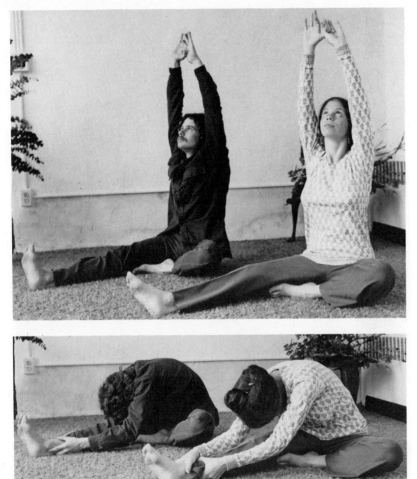

Extend the right leg to a 45-degree angle,
Bring the left foot to the inside of the right thigh,
Pull the foot in close to the body,
Lock thumbs, reach up, stretch . . .
Turn slightly to the right,

Exhale, drop over the right leg,
Hold onto the right leg, drop the head, the shoulders . . .
Relax . . .
Settle into the asana with every exhaling breath . . .
(1 minute)
and . . .
Lock thumbs, reach for the foot, stretch up!

Extend the left leg, pull the right foot in,
Lock thumbs, stretch up,
Turn to the left,

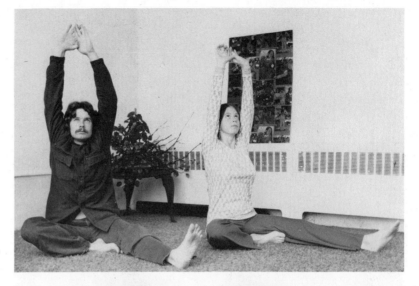

Exhale dropping down . . .
Hold onto the leg, drop the head, the shoulders . . .
Relax!
Settle into the pose with every exhalation . . .
(1 minute)
and . . .
Lock thumbs, stretch up,
Bring the feet together, stretch again . . .
Lower the back to the floor,
Stretch out on the floor
and
Savasana . . . relax . . . let go,
Watch the body, watch the breath. . . .

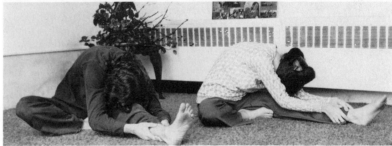

Spinal Twists (Arddha Matsyendrasana)

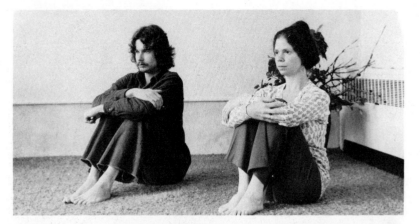

Bring the knees up to the chest,
Wrap the arms around the knees,
Push the head up toward the ceiling,

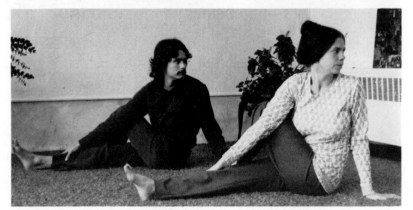

Extend the right leg, bring the left foot to the right side of the right knee,
Put the left hand behind the back, on the floor,
Extend the right arm and bring it to the left side of the left knee, have a grasp on the right knee,
Turn all the way to the left, chin even with the left shoulder . . .
(30 seconds)
and . . .

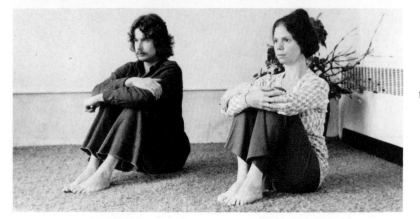

Bring the head around to the front,
Knees up to the chest,
Wrap the arms around the knees,
Push the head up,
Extend the left leg, bring the right foot to the left side of the left knee,
Put the right hand behind the back, on the floor,

56

Extend the left arm and bring it to the right side of the right knee, have a grasp on the left knee,

Turn all the way to the right, chin even with the right shoulder . . .

(30 seconds)

and . . .

Bring the head around to the front, knees up to the chest, wrap the arms around the knees, push the head up . . .

and . . .

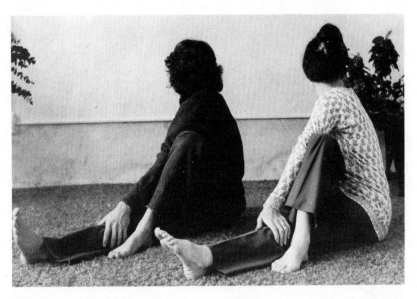

Stomach Lift with Pelvic Floor Contraction (Uddhiyana and Mula Bandha)

Sit in Vajrasana, buttocks resting on the heels,

Exhale forcefully through the mouth, close mouth,

Drop the head slightly . . . do not inhale!

Pull in the abdominal wall, all the way back toward the spine,

Pull up on the anal sphincter . . .

(Hold for 15 seconds)

Use a constant but not too strong pressure,

Relax the abdomen and sphincter,

Inhale, raise the head,

Repeat twice.

The Bandhas, when done with the breath exhaled, give a massage to all the internal organs, while firming the muscles of the lower abdomen and the pelvic floor.

The Bandhas, when done with the breath inhaled, focus the prana (vital force) at certain points (cakras) along the spine.

The locks help the prana to function as a unified force, increasing concentration and centering.

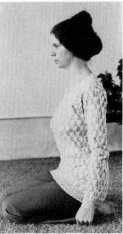
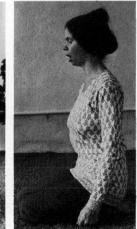
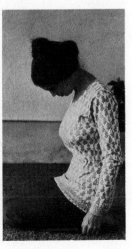

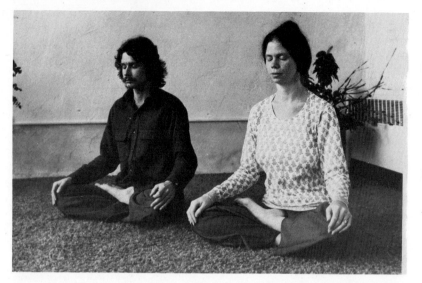

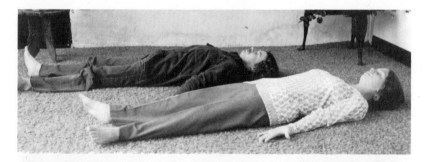

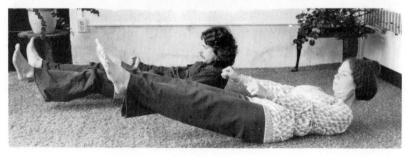

Bellows Breathing (Kapalabhati)

Kapalabhati is a series of forceful exhalations produced by pulling in the belly. Between every exhale there is an inhale, but unlike the exhale (which is forced), the inhale is relaxed.

This exercise should be done with speed. After the *quick* forceful exhale, *inhale immediately* and *quickly!*

Sit in a comfortable cross-legged position or half-lotus pose (left foot on right thigh, right foot under left thigh).

Exhale completely! Inhale fully and begin . . . pull in just the belly, force out some air . . . relax, inhale . . .

pull in the belly . . . relax . . .

pull in . . . relax . . .

pull in . . . relax . . .

Continue for about 40 expulsions, which constitutes one round. After each round take a few deep breaths, then relax and watch the breath, observing the effects after each round.

Do three rounds.

Quick Relaxation

Savasana . . . let go . . .
Now stretch out, push the hands away, feet away, and
Inhale! Full tension,
Raise the body . . . hold it . . .
Exhale! Drop!
Roll the legs and arms . . . relax . . . let go . . .

Tense the buttocks . . . relax,
Inhale, push out the belly . . .
Exhale! Mouth wide open!
Inhale, push out the chest . . .
Exhale, wide open mouth,
Squeeze the shoulders up . . . relax,

Push the face up . . . relax,
Stretch the face, open the mouth wide, eyes wide open,
push the tongue out . . . relax,
Roll the head back and forth . . .
Relax . . . let go.

Let the body go, part by part . . .
Starting with the feet, let the feet relax . . .
and ankles and calves . . .
Let the knees and thighs relax . . .
Now the hands and wrists . . .
The forearms, upper arms . . .
Let the whole trunk relax . . .
First the lower trunk (buttocks and lower
abdomen) . . .
Then the middle . . .
Finally the upper (chest and upper back) . . .
The whole trunk should feel as if it's sinking into the
floor . . .

Now the shoulders . . . let go . . .
The neck and throat . . .
The face . . . all the facial muscles are slack . . .
Even the top of the head . . .

The whole body . . . completely let go . . .

Watching the breath . . .
The more you watch it, the slower it goes . . .
Every time the mind wanders, bring it back to the
breath. . . .
(3 to 5 minutes)

WHEN YOU HAVE IT
GOING

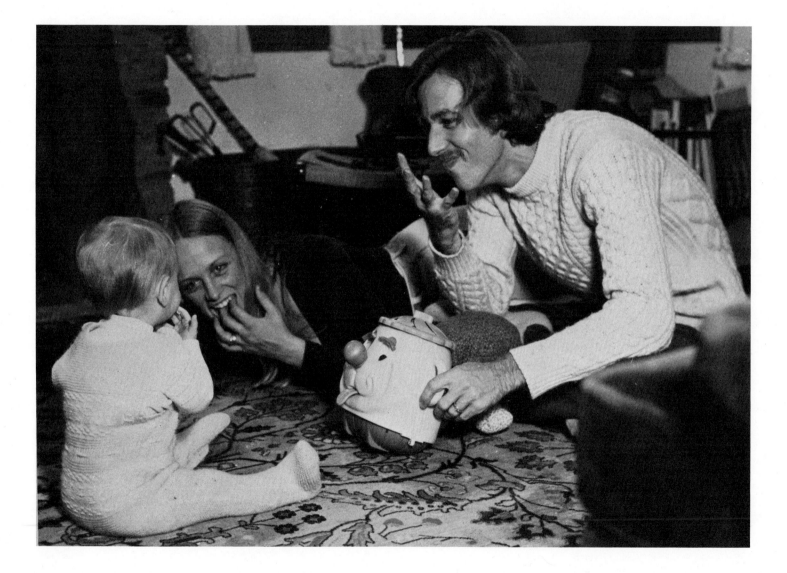

After a few months, the baby has established some kind of schedule.

Schedule yourself!

Find a particular time of day, every day, to do your yoga.

Be gentle with yourself, don't push,

Consistency will come as you relax into the practice.

CAUTION: *Do not do any inverted postures until six weeks after giving birth!*

Cobra (Bhujangasana)

Bring the palms under the shoulders, elbows pointing up,

Have the feet together, toes pointing back,

Put the forehead on the floor.

Begin the asana by stretching out the chin and tilting the head all the way back,

Use the muscles of the lower back to raise the shoulders and upper trunk from the floor,

Apply pressure on the palms, arching the back,

Roll the eyes all the way up, looking toward the ceiling . . .

Hold it, but don't tense!

Relax into the pose, let the spine arch, let the body settle into it with every exhale . . .

(1 minute)

Slowly come down . . .

Keep the chin extended until it touches the floor, then bring the forehead to the floor and

Return to Savasana . . . relax. . . .

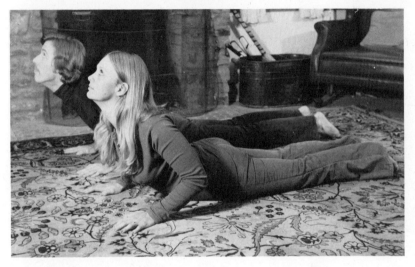

Locust Pose (Salabasana)

As in half-locust,
Bring the arms underneath the body,
Chin on the floor, feet together,
and
Raise both legs, keeping them straight,
Don't hold the breath,
Hold for 30 seconds . . .
and
Slowly lower the legs,
Bring the arms out . . .
Savasana . . . relax. . . .

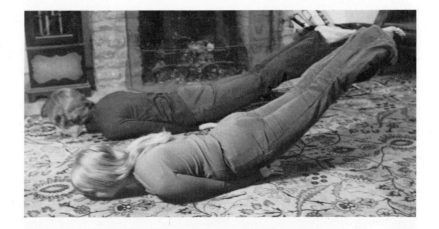

Bow Pose (Dhanurasana)

Bend the legs and have a grasp on the feet or ankles,
Bring the forehead to the floor,
and
Stretch out the chin,
Tilt the head back, look up,
Push the feet away (gently) as if you were trying to
straighten the legs,
Arch the spine,
Keep the feet together,
Don't hold the breath!
Relax with every exhale . . .
Relax into the asana, don't strain!
If it's comfortable, gently rock in the position . . .
(1 minute)
Slowly coming down . . .
Keep the chin extended,
Bring the chin to the floor,
Now forehead to the floor
and
Let go of the feet . . .
and
Savasana . . . relax!

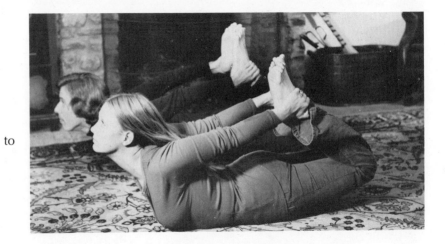

63

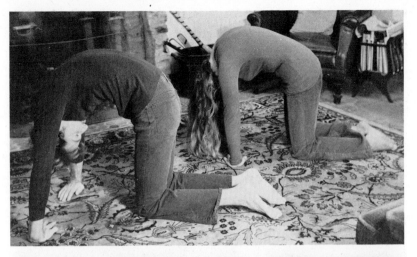

Cat and Cow

Standing on the hands and knees, fingers pointing toward each other,
Exhale! Drop the head, push the back up!

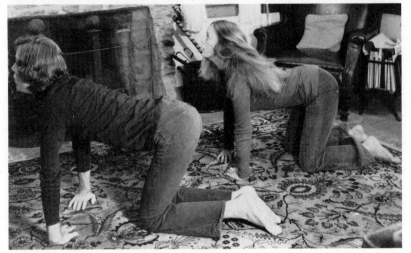

Inhale, pull the head back and arch the spine toward the floor . . .
Exhale . . . drop . . . push the back up,
Inhale . . . pull up the head . . . sway the back . . .
Continue . . . Exhale . . . Inhale . . .
(ten times)
Savasana on the back. . . .

Full Forward Bending (Paschimothanasana)

Arms overhead, lock thumbs . . . stretch! . . .
and

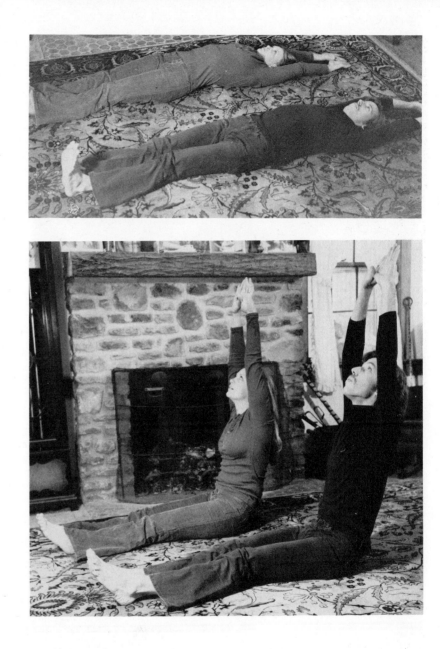

Sit up, stretch for the ceiling . . .

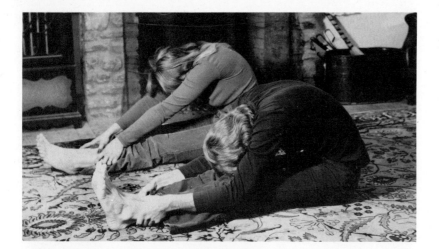

Exhale, dropping all the way down . . .
Relaxing into it . . .
(3 minutes)
and
Lock thumbs, reach for the feet . . .
Stretch up . . .
and

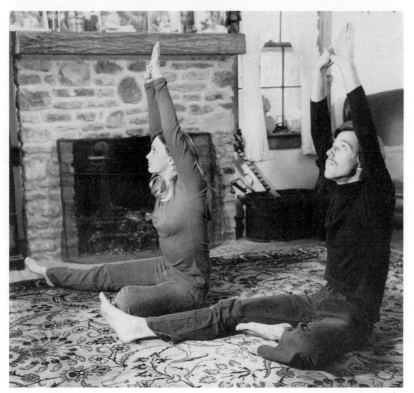

Head-to-Knee Pose (Janu-Sirs Asana)

Extend the right leg,
Left foot in . . .
Stretch up . . . turn right,

Exhale coming down . . .
(Hold 2 minutes)
and
Lock thumbs, stretch for the feet,
Reach up . . .
Extend the left leg,
Pull the right foot in . . .
Stretch . . . turn left,
Exhale coming down . . .
(2 minutes)
and
Lock thumbs, reach for the feet . . .
Stretch up . . .
Feet together . . .
Lower the back to the floor . . . Stretch . . .
and
Savasana . . . relax. . . .

The Wheel Pose (Cakrasana)

Place the palms flat on the floor, under the shoulders,
fingertips pointing toward the feet,
Feet flat on the floor, knees bent,
Push with the hands and feet until you can place the
top of the head on the floor,
Arch the back . . .
Only if comfortable, push still further, raising the head
off the floor,
Push the pelvis toward the ceiling . . .
(15 seconds)
and
Coming down . . .
Back on the floor,
Extend the legs, arms . . .
Savasana . . . relax. . . .

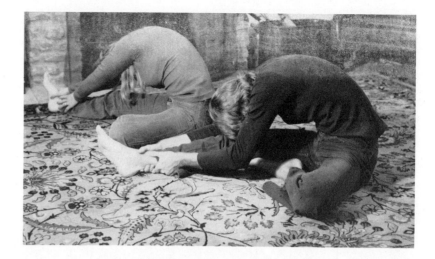

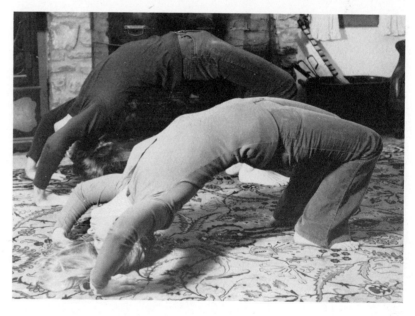

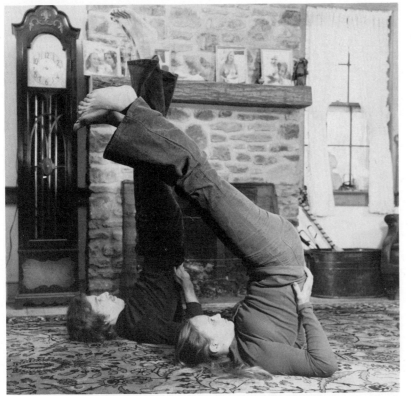

Shoulder Stand (Sarvangasana)

Bring the feet together,
Palms flat on the floor,
Raise the legs (keeping them straight) over the head, parallel to the floor,
Put the hands on the back,
Come to a vertical position, feet, hips, shoulders in one line . . .
Relax into it . . . let the weight settle on the shoulders and back of the neck.
If you can't get perfectly vertical, don't worry about it, just relax, don't strain . . .
(3 to 5 minutes)
Lower the legs overhead . . .
Roll the back down . . .
Keeping the legs straight, lower the feet to the floor . . .
Savasana . . . relax. . . .

The Fish Pose (Matsyasana)

Bring the feet together, palms under the thighs,
Arch the back, push the chest up,
Place the top of the head on the floor,
Hands on top of the thighs and . . .
Breathe deeply! Inhale all the way . . .
Exhale completely, pulling in the belly, forcing out all the air, and . . .
Inhale . . . Exhale . . .
Inhale . . . Exhale . . . (about ten times)
Let the breath return to normal . . .
Place the palms under the thighs,
Raise the head, lower the back to the floor,
Feet apart, Savasana . . . relax . . .
Watch the breath for 1 or 2 minutes and
Sit up . . .

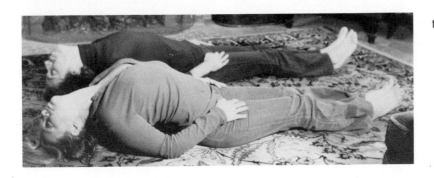

Spinal Twists (Arddha Matsyendrasana)

Knees to the chest,
Wrap the arms around the knees, push the head up . . .
and . . .
Bring the left foot under the right thigh,
Right foot to the left of the left knee,
Right hand on the floor behind the back,
Extend the left arm, bring it to the outside of the right knee,
Grasp the left knee,
Turn all the way to the right, chin even with the right shoulder, look back . . .

(15 seconds)
and . . .
Knees to the chest . . .
Arms around the knees, head up . . .
Right foot under the left thigh,
Left foot to the right of the right knee,
Left hand on the floor behind the back,
Extend the right arm, bring it to the outside of the left knee,
Grasp the right knee,
Turn all the way to the left, chin even with the left shoulder, look back . . .

(15 seconds)
and . . .
Knees to the chest, stretch up.

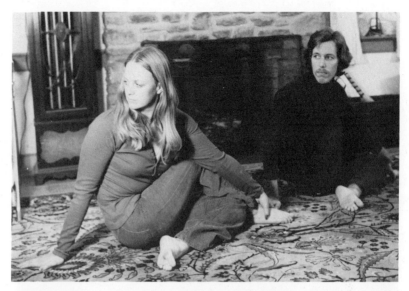

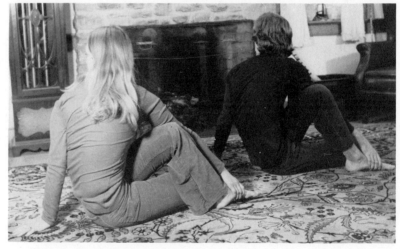

69

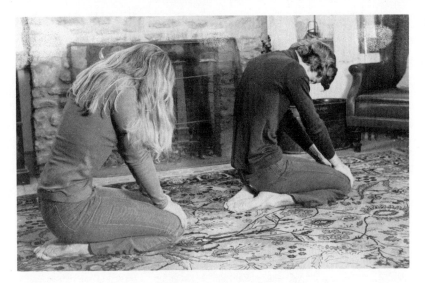

Stomach Lift with Pelvic Floor Contraction (Uddhiyana and Mula Bandha)

Sit in Vajrasana, hands on the knees,
Exhale (through the mouth),
Drop the head—don't inhale!—
Pull in the abdominal wall, pull up on the anal sphincter.
(Hold 15 seconds) (three times)

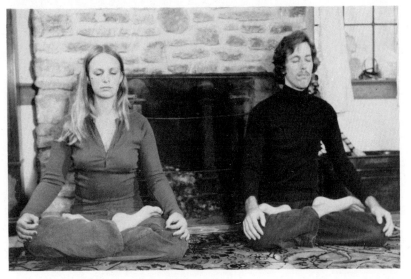

Bellows Breathing (Kapalabhati)

Sit in a meditative asana,
Exhale completely. . . . Inhale fully and
Begin. . . . Exhale just from the belly . . .
Inhale, relaxing the belly . . .
Exhale! Inhale!
Exhale! Inhale! . . .
(40 explusions.)

End with an exhale and . . .
Inhale deeply, hold it for a few seconds,
Exhale very slowly . . .
Let the breath return to normal,
Watch the breath for a moment.
(three rounds)

Alternate-Nostril Breathing (Nadi Shuddhi)

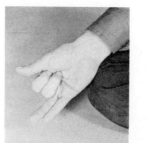

Sit in a meditative pose,

Hands on the knees,

Make a fist with the right hand, extend thumb, little and ring fingers,

Bring the hand to the face and close off the right nostril with the thumb,

Exhale from the left, empty the lungs completely . . .

Inhale from the left, use the three-part breathing . . . expand the belly, ribs, upper chest . . .

Close off the left with the little and ring fingers,

Slowly exhale from the right (from the chest, ribs, belly). . . .

Inhale from the right, close off the right with the thumb . . .

Exhale left . . .

Inhale left, close off the left with the little and ring fingers . . .

Exhale right . . .

Inhale right . . .

Switch nostrils, exhale left, inhale left. . . .

Make the exhale last twice as long as the inhale.

For example, if you inhale to the count of five, the exhale should last ten counts.

This exercise can be done for a few minutes to half an hour.

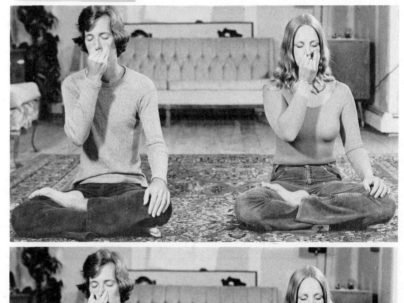

Meditation is simple or pure action. Pure as in something which is unalloyed with anything else, like pure sugar or pure gold. That is why, when the Buddha was asked what made him different from others, he said, "When hungry I just eat, when tired I just sleep."

Usually, when you do something, your mind is somewhere else, on something else. Rarely is it concentrated on the present, on the act you are performing at this moment; rather, the mind flits from recollections of the past to anticipation of the future.

Meditation is simple as opposed to our normal state of mind, which is complex, tense, filled with conflicting opinions, feelings, thoughts, and emotions. In short, we do not feel peaceful.

Meditation is the way to true peace as well as a direct expression of it.

If we were not inherently peaceful, there would be no way to become so! By practicing meditation we are not striving to become peaceful; rather, we're removing the mental restlessness which obscures our original, true nature of peace and happiness.

All beings possess this original, peaceful nature, but because of our conditioning, just the opposite appears to be true.

The yogic process is a process of deconditioning or unlearning. The aim of all the yoga practices and techniques is simply to provide the ability just to eat when you eat and to sleep when you sleep. If you could do this, yoga and meditation practice would be unnecessary.

The sitting posture (asana) is the most effective way to arrive at pure action or meditation. It is not only a way to meditation, but *is* meditation if you are seated properly. When all the elements of the asana are present (spine erect, body steady and firm but relaxed, head, neck, and

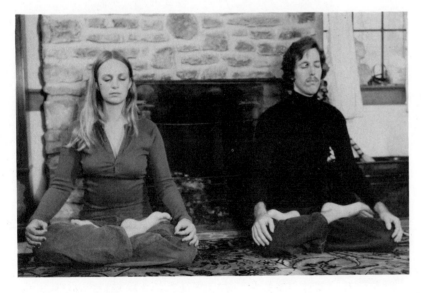

trunk in a straight line), the mind is concentrated.

Body posture is always synonymous with state of mind. That is why sitting is so difficult—it doesn't match your mental state, so it feels uncomfortable.

After some practice, sitting becomes easier, then enjoyable, as the mind arrives at steadiness.

Meditation Instructions

Sit in a meditative pose . . . back straight . . . the rest of the body relaxed . . . eyes closed!

Take full, deep breaths . . . remember! Use the three parts to breathe . . . inhale from the belly . . . exhale from the chest . . . continue for a few minutes. . . .

Let the breath come back to normal, don't control it! . . . just watch it . . . feel the breath flow in . . . feel it flow out . . . just keep following the breath with the mind . . . don't let your attention drift away! Every time it wanders, gently bring it back. . . . You will notice the breathing becoming slower and slower . . . this is a natural result of watching it.

You're not holding the breath; it just slows down by itself. You may also get some natural pauses between breaths. If the breath pauses, really focus the mind on the pause; this will be when the mind has the most steadiness and concentration. When thoughts come in to distract you, just let them go by . . . don't fight them . . . calmly, patiently bring the mind back to watching the flow of the breath. . . .

(Practice for a set length of time—10 to 15 minutes a day. As this becomes easier, gradually increase the time until sitting for one or two hours is no strain.)

. . . Take a few deep, full breaths . . .
Open the eyes, stretch out the legs. . . .

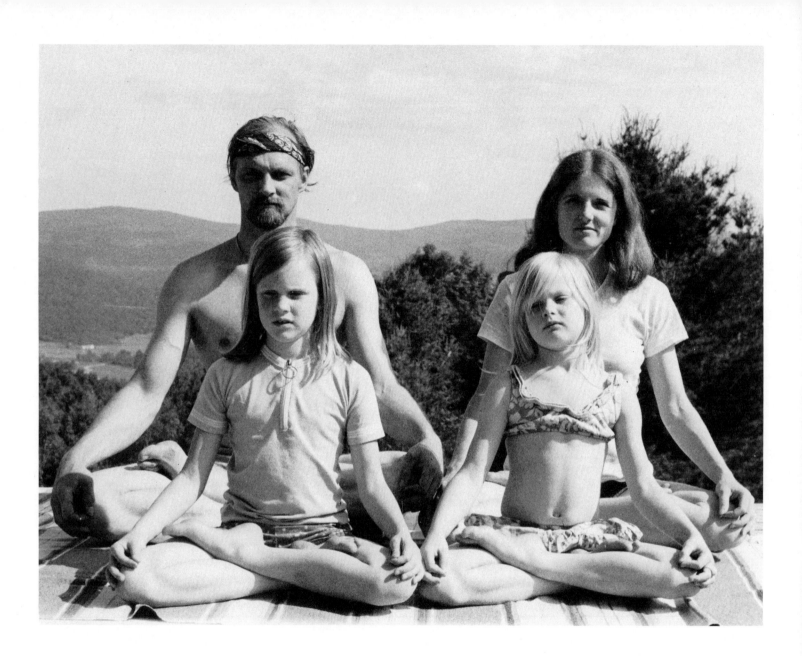

REGULAR PRACTICE

*If you lose the spirit of repetition, your
practice will become quite difficult.*

—*Shunryu Suzuki*
Zen Mind, Beginner's Mind

Note: Listed with each pose in this section are maximum
time limits—please don't exceed them. Make sure you
hold each pose only as long as comfortable (even if it's
only a fraction of the maximum time). Remember, don't
strain.

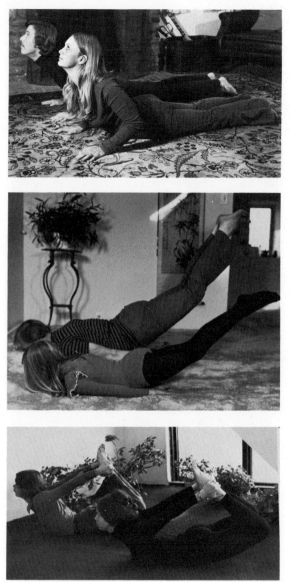

Cobra (Bhujangasana)

Palms under the shoulders, feet together, forehead on the floor . . .
Going up . . .
(1 minute)
Slowly coming down . . . keep the chin extended . . .
Savasana. . . .

Locust (Salabasana)

Arms underneath, chin on the floor . . .
Raising the legs . . .
(1 minute)
Savasana. . . .

Bow Pose (Dhanurasana)

Bend the legs, grasping the ankles . . . forehead on the floor . . .
Coming up . . .
Rock in the position . . .
(1 minute)
Turn over on the back . . . Savasana. . . .

Full Forward Bending (Paschimothanasana)

Remember,
Lock thumbs, stretch out, sit up, stretch up, then
Settle into it . . .
Let the head drop . . . sink into it . . .
Keep the mind on the body . . .
(1 minute)
If it's comfortable, and your elbows stay on the floor,
hook the index finger around the big toe, pulling the foot
back toward the head.
Lock thumbs, reach for the feet,
Stretch up and . . .

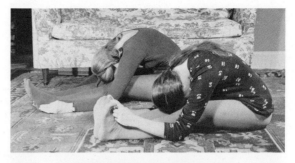

Head-to-Knee Pose (Janu-Sirs asana)

Extend the right leg,
If it's comfortable, place the foot on top of the thigh . . .
Relax with every exhale . . .
(2 minutes)
Extend the left leg . . .

Lock thumbs, reach for the feet, stretch up . . .
Bring the legs together . . .
Lower the back to the floor . . .
Savasana. . . .

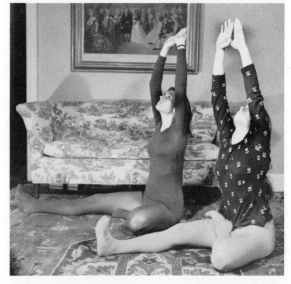

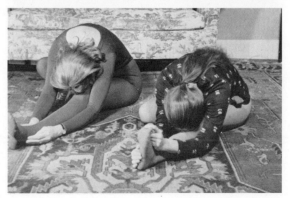

77

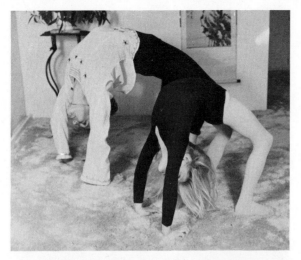

Wheel Pose (Cakrasana)

Push up . . .
Don't strain . . .
Gently walk the hands toward the feet . . .
Roll the back down . . .
(30 seconds)
Savasana. . . .

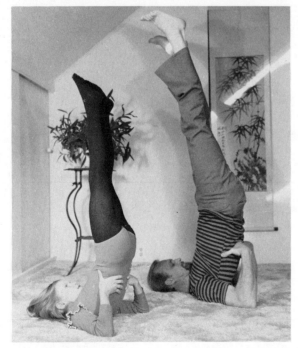

Shoulder Stand (Sarvangasana)

Palms on the floor,
Legs over the head,
Coming up . . .
Hands supporting back, let the weight settle on the shoulders and neck . . .
(up to 10 minutes)

Bridge Pose (Sethu Bandha Sarvangasana)

Another way to come out of the Shoulder Stand is by doing the Bridge Pose . . .
Keep the hands on the back,
Have one leg overhead, lower the other to the floor behind the back (not behind the head!),
Bring the other foot to the floor,
Keep the hands on the back and stretch the legs out . . .
Hold it . . .
And slide the elbows out, letting the back down . . .
Savasana. . . .

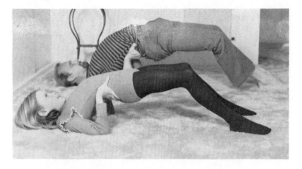

Fish Pose (Matsyasana)

Place the palms under the thighs,
Arch the back, place the top of the head on the floor,
Hands on top,
Deep breathing!
Arch the back all the way . . .
(2 minutes)
Raise the head, lower the back to the floor . . .
Savasana. . . .

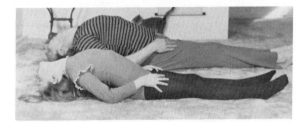

Spinal Twists (Arddha Matsyendrasana)

Sit up, knees to the chest, stretch up,
Left foot under right thigh,
Turn to the right,
Reach through the leg, grasp the hands behind the back
. . . hold . . .
and . . .
Stretch up . . .
Right foot under left thigh . . .
(1 minute each side)

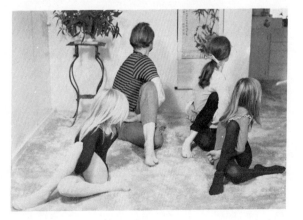

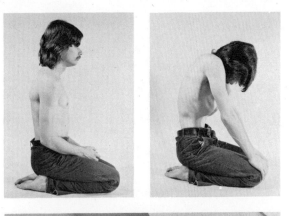

Stomach Lift with Pelvic Floor Contraction (Uddhiyana and Mula Bandha)

Air exhaled,
Pull in and up with a steady and firm (but not too hard) pressure . . .
(15 seconds)

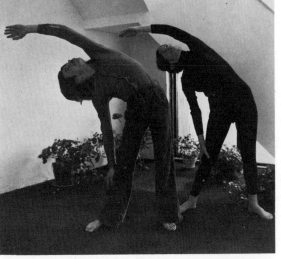

Triangle Pose (Trikonasana)

Stand with the feet apart (1 to 2 feet),
Arms outstretched parallel to the floor,
Turn the right palm up, left palm down,
and
Slowly lower the left hand to the side of the left leg,
Bring the right hand overhead,
Turn the head and look up at the right hand,
Slide the left hand as far down the leg as comfortable . . .
Hold for 30 seconds . . .
Coming up . . . arms parallel to the floor and . . .
Left palm up . . . right turned down . . .
and repeat, bending the body to the right.
(1 minute each side)

Pranayama with Breath Retention

Kapalabhati with retention is called *Bhastrika.*
After the last expulsion of each round, inhale deeply,
Hold the breath and lower the chin to the chest (this is called Jalandhra Bandha or the chin lock) . . .
Don't let the air leak out . . . hold as long as comfortable . . .

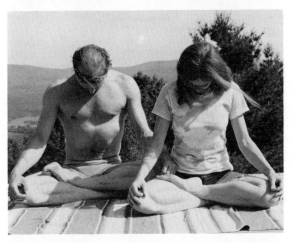

Raise the head and exhale as slowly as you possibly can, have a smooth exhale . . .
Let the breath come back to normal,
Watch the body and breath for a minute before starting the next round. . . .

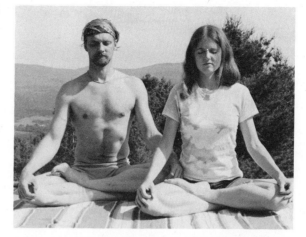

Nadi Shuddhi with retention is called *Sukha Purvika.* Retention of the breath should be added only when a 10:20 count is easy and comfortable. Begin by retaining the breath for a count of 5. The inhale would be 10 counts, hold for 5, then exhale for 20 counts. When this practice is easy and comfortable, raise the retention to 10 counts. The retention should be raised *slowly,* practicing each new ratio for weeks or months before increasing the holding count. In this way the retention is raised to 40 counts, making the pranayama last for 10 seconds on the inhale, 40 on the retention, and 20 on the exhale. Only raise the retention count when the previous ratio can be done for half an hour without strain!

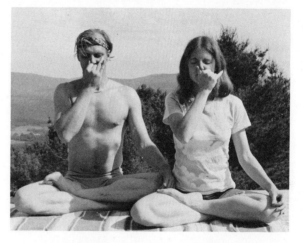

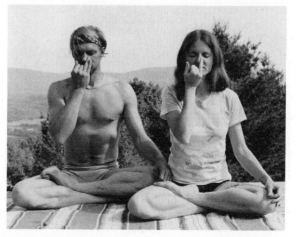

81

After pranayama just let the breath return to normal . . .
Don't control it! . . .
Watch the breath slow down. . . .

Now shift your attention to the mind,
Starting the meditation on the mind itself . . .
Just watch each thought one by one. . . .

As each thought arises, just observe . . .
Don't get caught up in it, don't judge it, don't think
discursively, this is good, that is bad, etc. . . .
You're not controlling anything, just seeing what is. . . .

The purpose of mind watching is *realizing* the watcher
(the Self—you!) is not the mind . . .
Even thoughts like "I am not the mind," "I am the
observer to the mind," are just more mental modifications
which arise and subside. . . .

EXPERIENCE

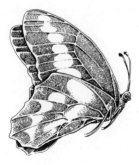

PARENTHOOD

"It's an adjustment!"

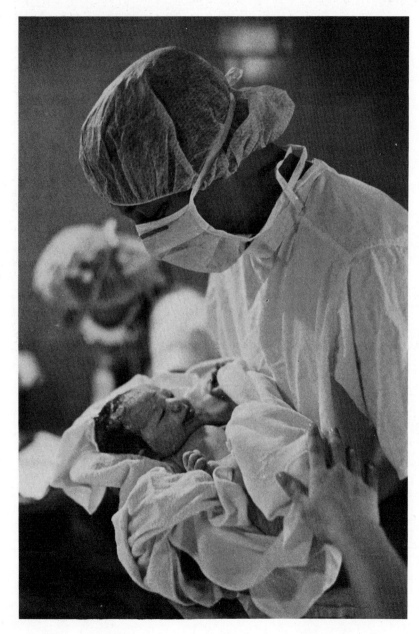

No matter how hard one has tried to prepare for parenthood, the reality is always a new and unexpected experience.

For the mother, birth and death meet at the moment when her baby takes his first independent breath. The being with whom she was one is now a separate individual—the joint self dies. In the first few months following birth, she and her child will be closely knit, but as the baby grows and develops he will become less and less dependent on her. She must learn to sense when to hold on, when to let go.

The father may find the first few weeks after birth difficult as he tries to help and support a woman whose full attention and energy are being spent on their child. Euphoric as he may be after the birth, the newborn infant and mother have a symbiotic relationship he cannot experience.

The male's exclusion is being minimized as more and more men become involved with the being and care of their infants. This is enriching for both male and female. The male is given an opportunity to express maternal tendencies and emotions that are a meaningful and very real part of his personality; the woman is given relief from her consuming involvement with the baby and from the heavy caretaking responsibilities of the first few weeks.

When my wife had to have a Caesarean section, I felt gypped. I'd been so much a part of everything up until then that I wanted to see the baby born. I think if I'd pushed harder the doctor would have let me into the operating room. When I talked to him afterward, he promised me that I could be there next time.
When the pediatrician brought the baby up from the operating room, he took me into the nursery with him. Both he and the nurse were wonderful. They told me everything they were doing. I really looked at the baby, and she looked at me.

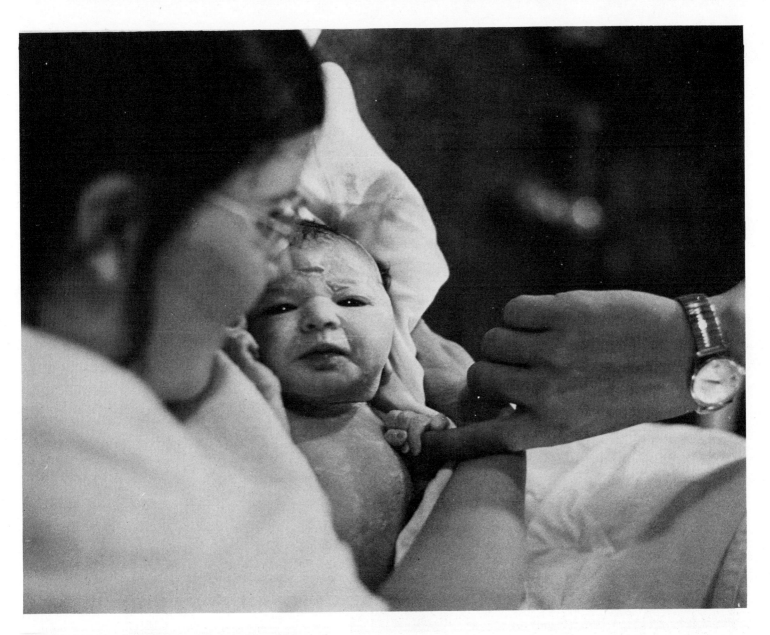

It came over me when she was minutes old and I looked into her eyes . . . that's a person! A whole, other person, not a carbon copy of one of us, but a whole human being.

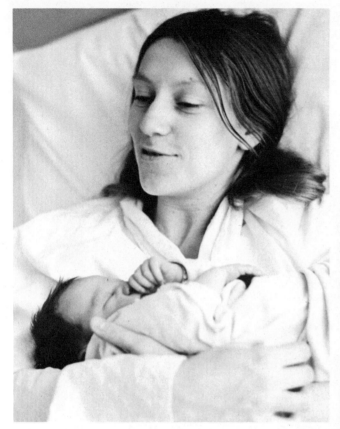

I wasn't sure if I just wanted to be pregnant or if I wanted to have a baby. As soon as I saw him, I felt relieved.

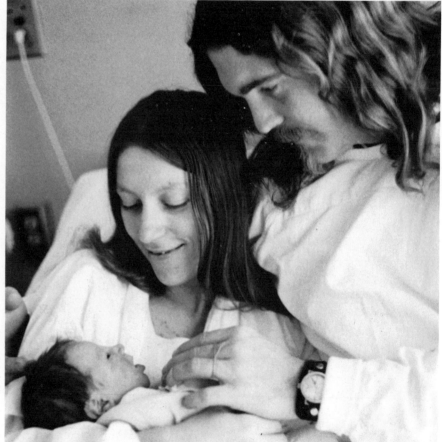

I didn't feel anything—just numb—until I went out for breakfast. When I came back and walked into the room, and she and the baby were there, it just came over me—a feeling of wonder that that person was a combination of the two of us. It's brought us closer together.

88

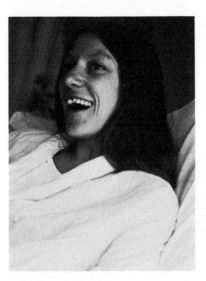

Everyone I talked to today, I told them it was the most beautiful thing I'd ever seen. They all said, "Would you go through it again?" I said, "Yes, I would, and the same way. I wouldn't miss it and I know Don wouldn't. He was so euphoric, just unreal. He was so excited, so happy."

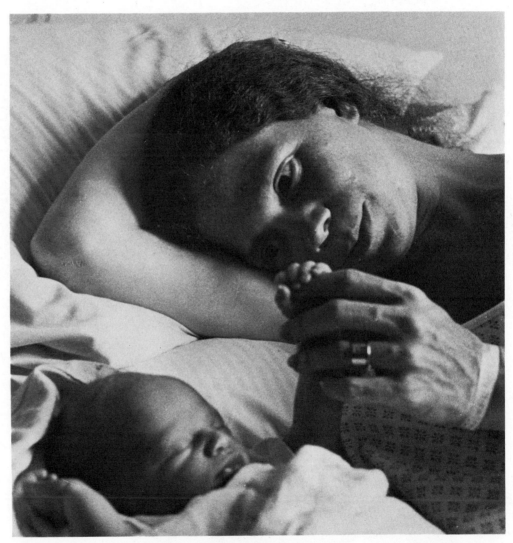

It's impossible to realize that he's here . . . that he was in my stomach just a few hours ago. I can't believe that such a perfectly formed being was in there.

89

The awareness that one is a *parent* comes slowly. Sometimes it hits in all-encompassing flashes, sometimes it is forgotten, sometimes the awareness of the responsibilities brings stabs of anxiety. Overall, it is a slow, ever expanding identification of oneself with a new and very different role.

It all dawned on me when I began to realize I would have to care for a child for so many years.

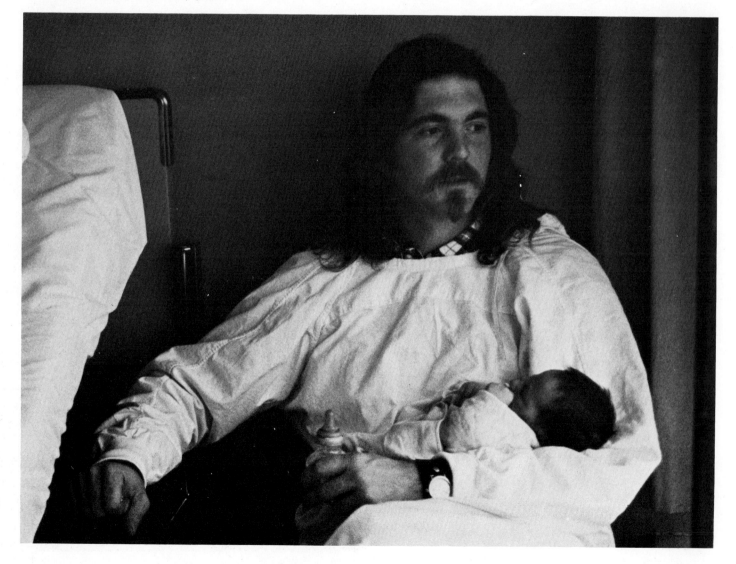

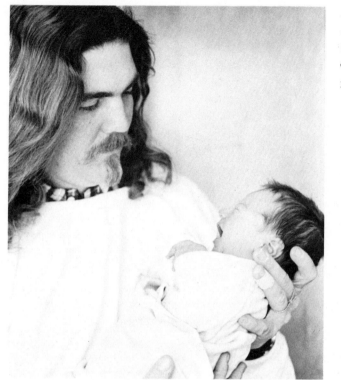

I keep flashing back to my childhood, remembering bits and pieces. The giant who would pick me up and touch me to the ceiling or take me fishing or play catch on rare occasions. How I loved him! Still do, but from an adult point of view.

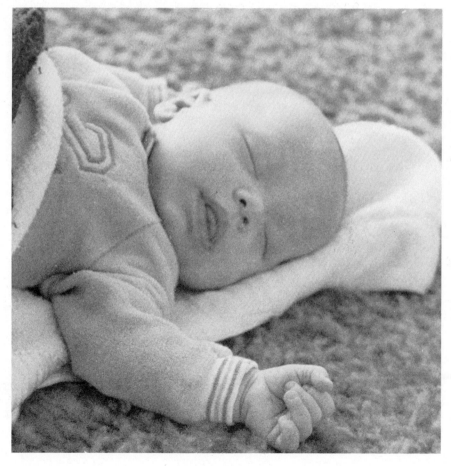

The first day we brought the baby home we left him in the living room. I went to sleep in my room, and when I woke up and he wasn't there, I thought I'd lost him. It really gave me a scare.

I didn't really have postpartum depression. But I would have crying spells. I think it was wonder. I was so awed that that was my baby lying there that I would burst into tears.

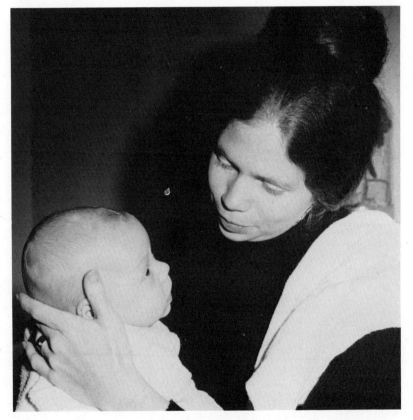

The first few days after birth are often euphoric. Many parents are infused by a sense of wonder and triumph at having participated in a primal experience. But there is also the awareness that the moment of the peak experience is past. Now one must begin to adjust to a new state of being, to a relationship, involving heavy caretaking responsibilities, with another person—a stranger.

For the mother, physical changes make an already tenuous emotional state more difficult. Suddenly her great stomach is gone, no one lives there now but her intestines and organs, which are slowly finding their usual places and resuming their nonpregnant level of function. Stretch marks, loose skin, blood emptying from an unoccupied uterus, bruised tissues, and soreness are lingering reminders of the cataclysmic event that brought her child into the world. Soon her swelling breasts and the presence of milk will bring her to a full awareness that, separate though they are, she and her child are still very dependent on each other.

She may wish someone would mother her, and here she is—faced with *being* a mother and supposed to know—by some magic often beyond her—*how* to do it! It's a difficult time!

Having him in the room with me when I was in the hospital made it much easier when I got home. I was already used to taking care of him.

92

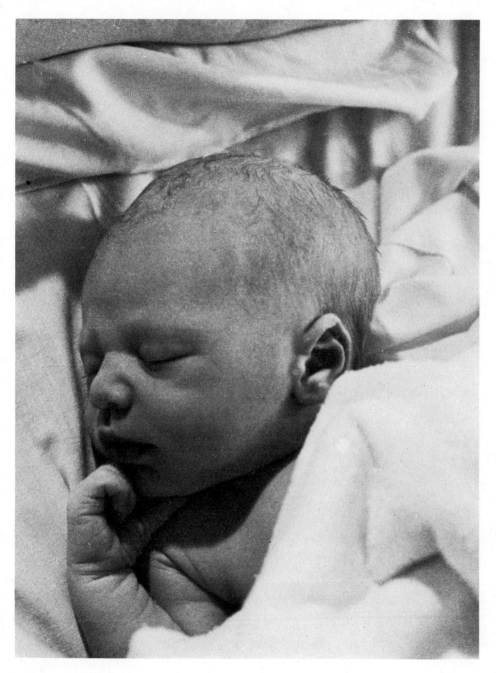

I had a dream that the baby was lying in the car bed. I heard him making little noises and I felt guilty that I wasn't checking on him. But I kept telling myself: You don't have to watch him every minute. When I went over, his head was in a pan of water—one of the kitchen pots— completely submerged, but he was fine, breathing and everything.

93

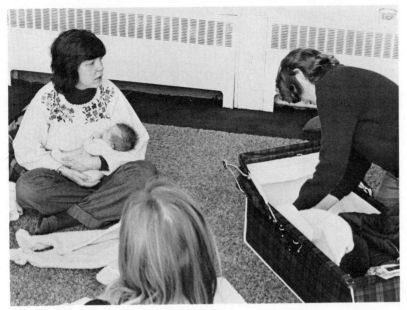

Now, *anytime you go anywhere, there's* stuff! *I used to just go—not anymore. I spent an hour today looking for the car keys. I'd put them on top of the car while I was loading all the junk.*

I can't believe how much work it is! I keep thinking: No one ever told me that so much was going to be demanded of me.

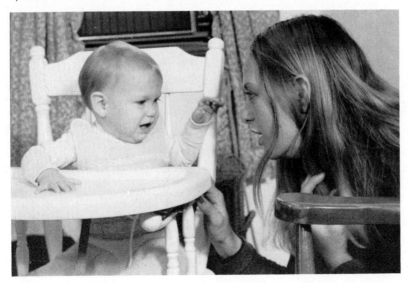

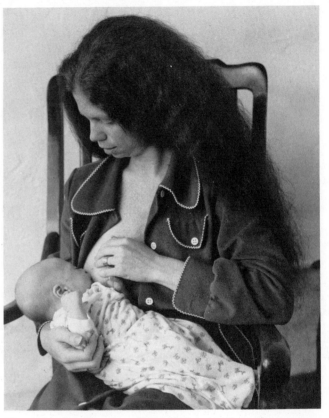

He eats a lot! It seems like all the time!

When you don't sleep, everything is all one thing. It's been one continuous day since she was born.

94

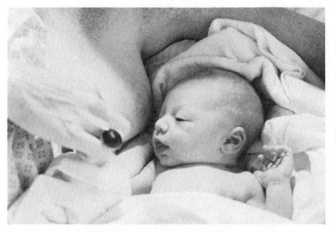

I had a dream that my baby was just a head, a huge head. He was lying next to another baby who had arms and legs. They told me it was all right, that at a certain age they have the arms and legs sewn on. I looked at the other baby, trying to see where his arms and legs had been sewn on, but I couldn't.
I guess it's the head that's important at this stage; the rest of the body doesn't become important until later.
Actually, I guess I see the baby as one big mouth.

Her daily activities change. Baby care absorbs much more time and effort than most people expect. Babies don't understand schedules and organization. They have no empathy for a tired or depressed mother.

The woman who tends to operate on an abstract level is often the mother who suffers the most when reality and anticipation don't meet.

The trick is to let go . . . to surrender to the experience . . . to let it happen. Suddenly there is joy in the moment, in this special state of being, in this unique happening. . . .

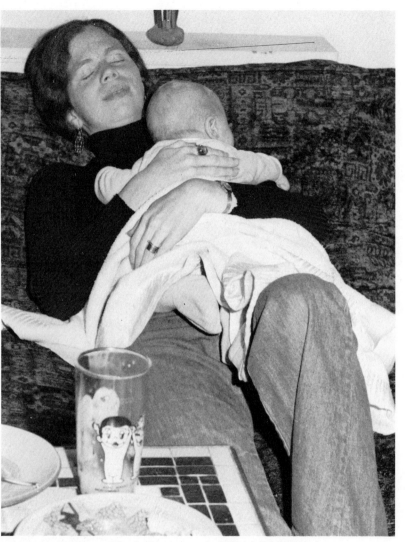

I had pictured myself naked, on top of a hill, child at my breast, hair blowing in the wind. It was hard to adjust to reality!

95

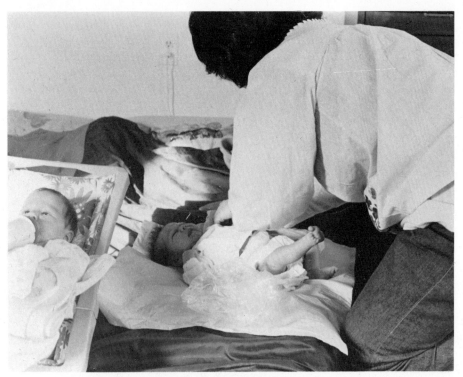

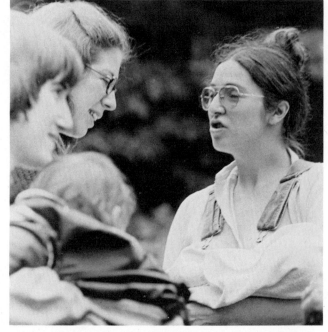

When I was pregnant, I was afraid I wouldn't be able to change diapers. I had a girl friend who had a baby, and every time she was changing a diaper or the baby threw up, I'd gag. It started to freak me.

The first six weeks nearly drove me crazy. It seemed as if I'd just put him down and there would be that little voice again. "Oh, no," I'd say. "Baby, I just fed you!"

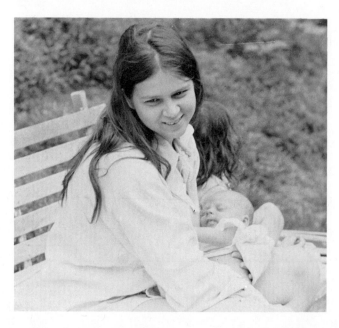

I feel so protective—whenever I take the baby out in the carriage and people peer into it, I feel like covering him with my body and shooing them away.

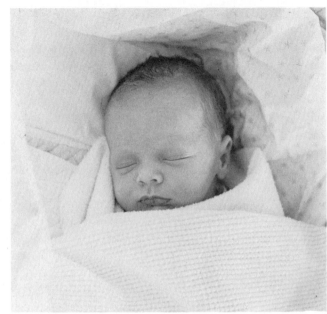

It got so when I looked at my husband's face, it seemed huge! I spend so much of my time staring at that tiny face that my husband seems like a giant!

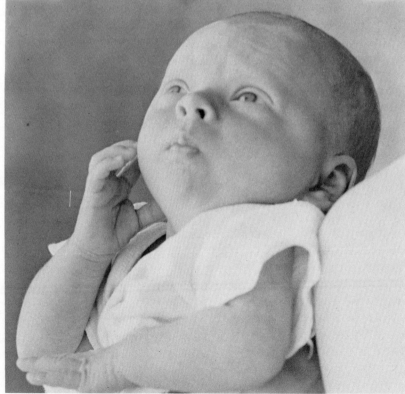

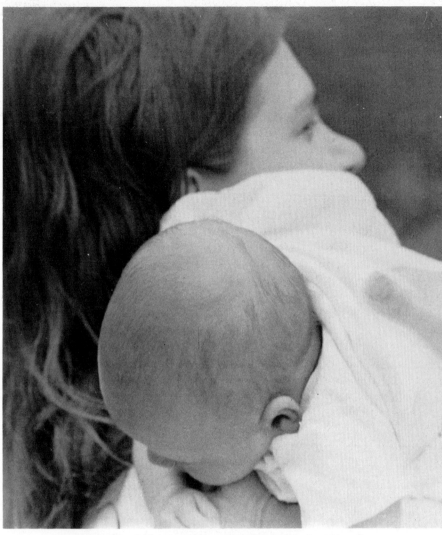

I was so blasé about the nursing that when he started having colic, and people told me it could be from my own tension, I was really surprised.
After that I started noticing the times when he spit up or seemed tense, and they were often related to the times when I was tense or anxious.

And, along with it all, is her own status. One of the first things most mothers do when they get home from the hospital is to stand nude in front of a mirror to assess the situation. For a new mother, it may be a shock to see how much her body has changed. Despite the way it looks the first week or two after giving birth, the stomach—with a little effort—will be flat again. The changed shape of the breasts, the stretch marks—faded to white traces—are there to stay. She now has a mother's body, a body that has fulfilled its function and has reached maturity.

Sex, in the first few weeks after birth, may be difficult. Different doctors advise varying lengths of abstinence. During any period of abstinence, sexual inventiveness helps. But often fatigue, soreness, and lack of interest make the woman a less than enthusiastic sex partner. The nursing mother may find her usual lubrication failing her (use a lubricant!), and orgasm may bring a gush of milk from her breasts. Some men like it, others don't.

Mechanical problems can be dealt with; the biggest obstacles are fatigue and the nervous anticipation that the baby may cry at any minute and demand attention. Try having childless friends babysit while you go to *their* apartment for a "just the two of us" orgy!

The end of the first six weeks usually brings relief and perspective. Many babies drop one feeding at about this time. Five or six hours of solid sleep can feel like pure heaven. A frayed sense of humor may suddenly be fresh and alert. And, best of all, after all that effort on the parents' part, the baby starts to respond! A small but very significant reward for all that has been given.

As the baby begins to be more regular of habit, and as the mother is less fatigued, life becomes more orderly. Now, in addition to the emotional aspects of being parents, the organizational aspects can be dealt with.

The woman has had some time to reflect on her new role, to experience herself as a mother. She begins to feel her way toward the kind of person she will be and the kind of life she will lead as a mother.

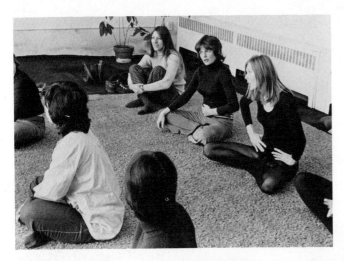

I was amazed at how long it took my stomach to get flat.
Right after I had the baby, I still looked pregnant.
I feel so fat! I just want to lose weight!

Doing yoga until late in the pregnancy made a big
difference. I could do all the exercises they gave me in the
hospital with no effort at all.

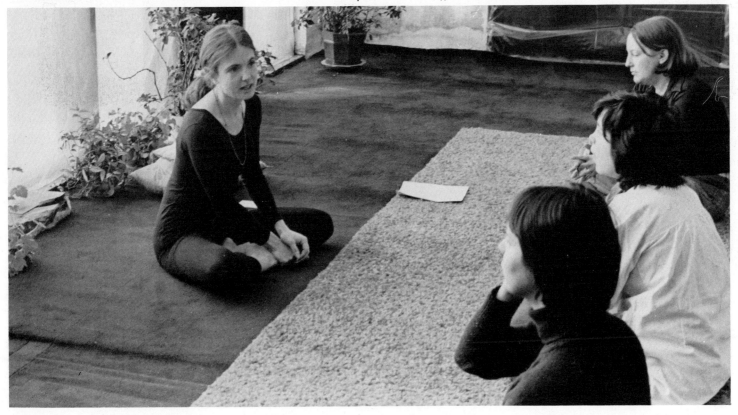

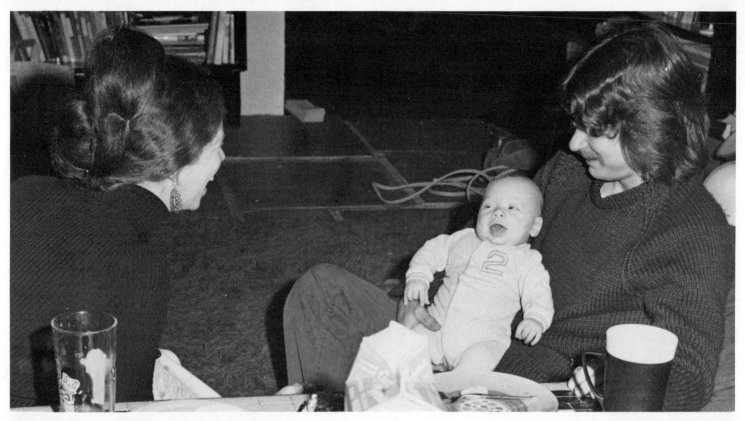

When he first smiled, that's the nicest thing that's happened. It's so beautiful to see a baby smiling. You want to know that the baby's comfortable, that he's happy, and there's no way of knowing until he smiles. It's a recognition of you, too.

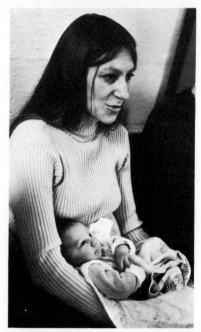

I wasn't going to let the baby change my life. Then you come to the realization that, with the baby feeding every hour, you can't run out anytime you want, and even if you could, you're too tired.

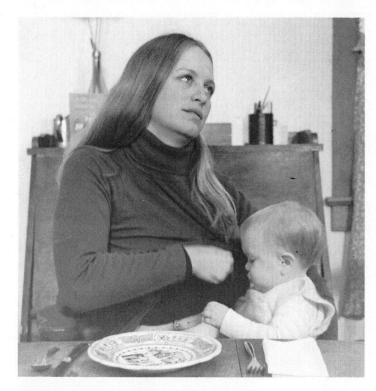

I started doing things right away. I'd made up my mind that having a baby wasn't going to stop me. I took her everywhere with me. I don't think it would have been that way if I hadn't been nursing. That made it much easier.

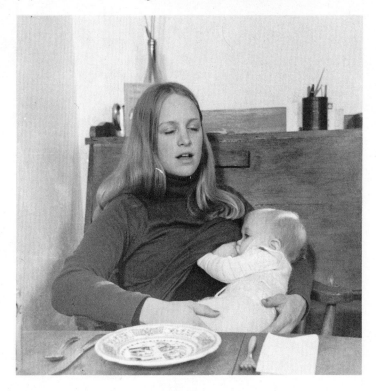

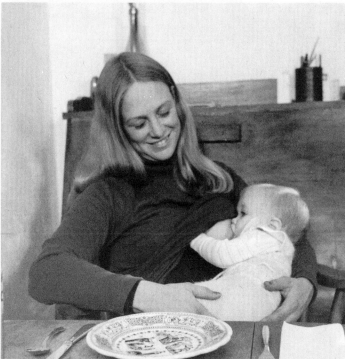

If you want to do something, you'll find a way. If you let the baby make you feel tied down, if you restrict yourself, you tend to blame the baby, to feel resentment. I'd rather have someone else watch her than start building up resentment.

101

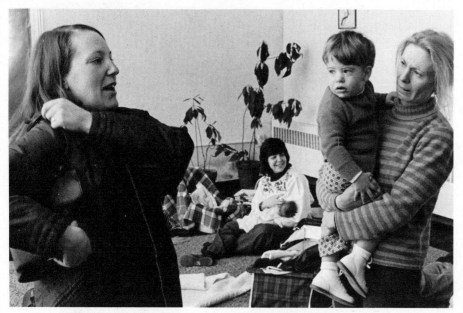

It helps to talk with other people. I thought I'd have it much better organized than this. It's nice to know I'm not the only one who can't seem to get it together.

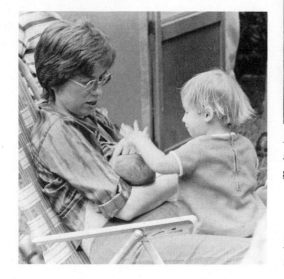

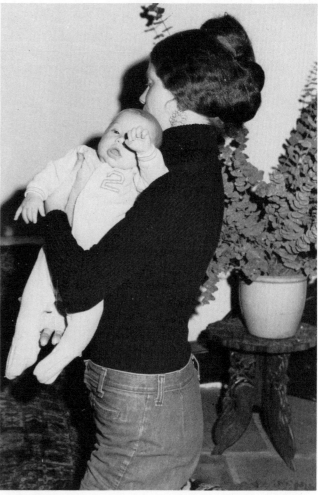

I can listen to the crying for a while, but then it really starts to get to me. There's a special sound to it that just gets you!

I sometimes resent other people for not understanding how much it takes out of me to care for the children.

As their world focuses on BABY, the father may be the least cared-for member of the group. He can't experience the physical bond that is between mother and baby, but he is expected to understand, to involve himself with the infant, to help the mother, and to provide for all of them.

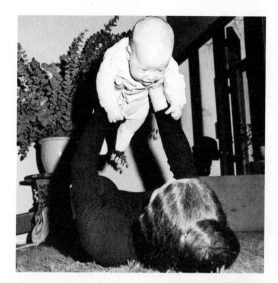

The biggest thrill is realizing they're coming to know you.

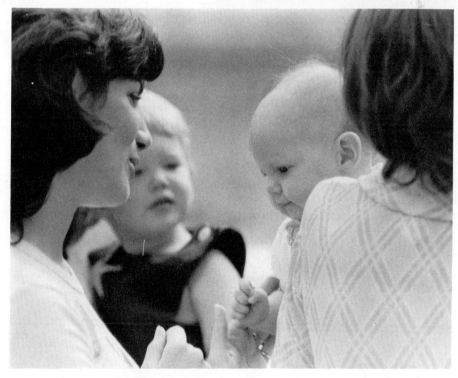

The male is bound to be left out to some extent. Look at how the hormones are affected by breast feeding. There's so much going on biologically between mother and baby that just can't happen between the father and the baby.

My focus was much different than my wife's. I was aware of the baby's being there in terms of responsibility, not as a close physical bond.

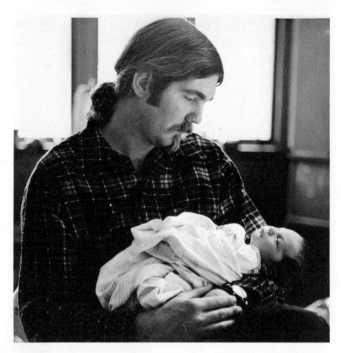

From the beginning, there's no contest. Even at the birth, mother and baby are there together, you're just standing there.
She says she wishes you were more involved, but when you see them together, and see all the baby's needs being met, you feel almost useless, except as you can contribute to the mother's well-being, helping her to be able to do her thing better.

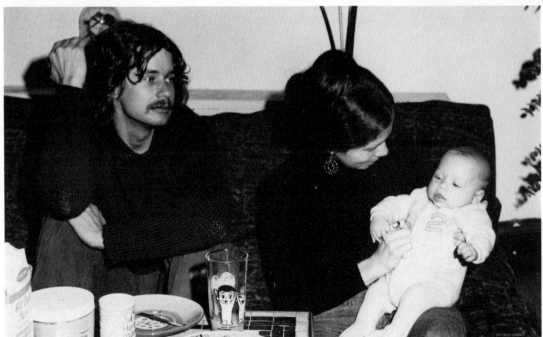

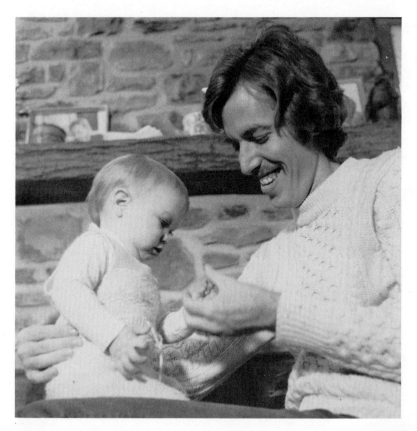

At the beginning, all I could do was to help my wife. I couldn't get really physically close to the baby until she began to know me. It all happened at once. One night I walked by her crib—and she screamed bloody murder that I hadn't spoken to her.

We used to do everything together. After the baby, we began doing things separately. I don't think it's bad—it's just brought us to a new part of our lives. I finally had to decide that I was going to work, to make decisions about the structure of my life.

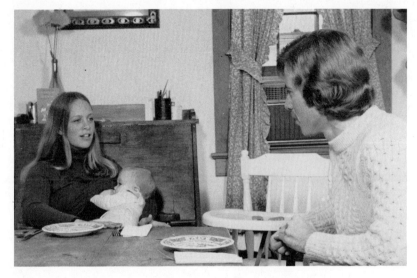

The couple's relationship changes. At the most basic level, there is another person in the house. They are no longer lovers and alone, but are parents as well. Their existing roles don't disappear, but new roles and responsibilities are added. The adjustment takes time.

A troubled relationship is further stressed. There isn't time to work things out, to be with each other, to get into one another. Responsibilities seem greater, obstacles more insurmountable, when they are faced by the individual rather than by the couple as a unit.

A strong relationship holds firm more easily. The stresses of parenthood bring more laughter than rage and tears. The joy in the child comes from each of the individuals and from the couple as a unit.

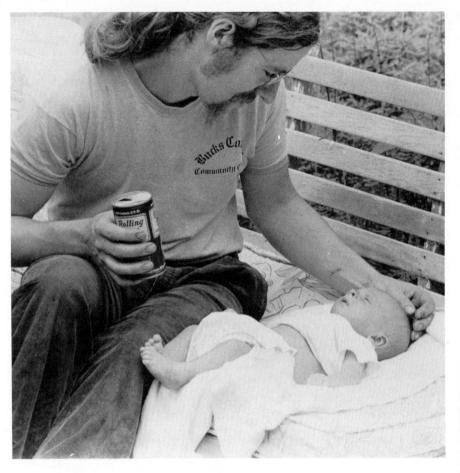

I didn't go through any anxiety or pain—I just noticed that my beer consumption doubled.

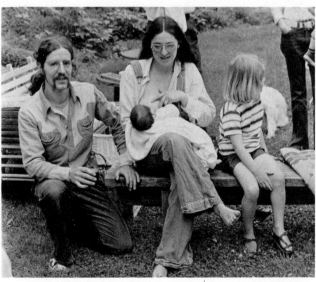

Things haven't been nearly as hard as I expected they would be. Maybe because this baby wasn't planned we dreaded the actuality. We had fears of having to give up our life style, of all kinds of changes in our lives. The actual presence of the baby alleviated all those fears—it wasn't the end of the world!

106

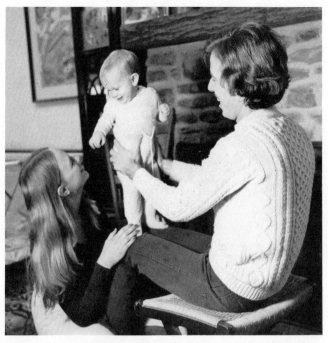

All of a sudden there's a link between two people—something more than the two of you. I feel as if I'm with my wife and the baby all day long, even if I'm not. I don't know if it's because the baby is part of me, but I don't feel separated. It's brought us closer mentally—not exactly mentally—maybe spiritually.

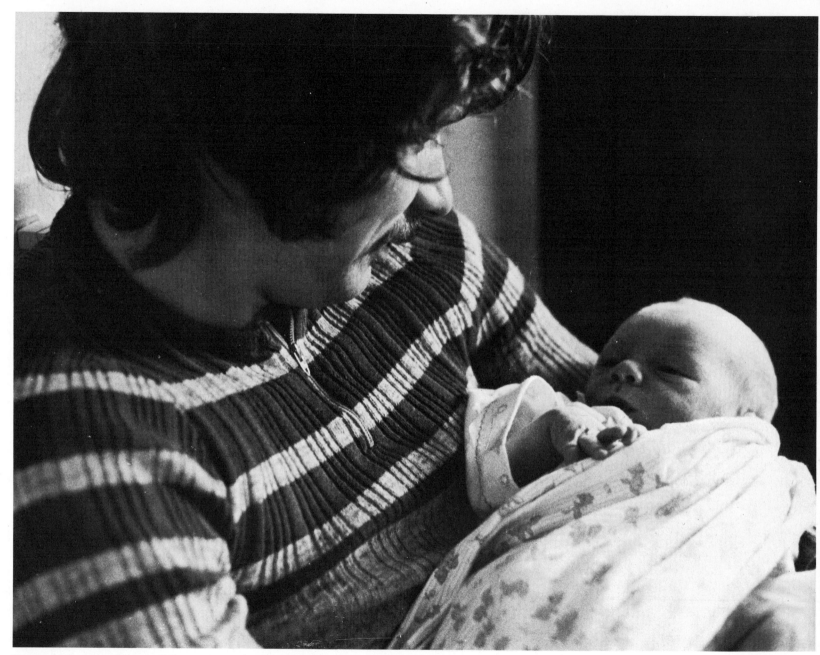

Your relationship changes, it has to, now there's a third person, a third part of you.

It's a bigger burden for the mother than for the father. I can always go out and go to work. I can understand the wife getting uptight. But she should understand that I'm doing something that has to be done too.

Sometimes I felt the baby came before me. But I knew that was the way it should be. It's a matter of understanding that the feeling is there—it would be absurd to get uptight about it.

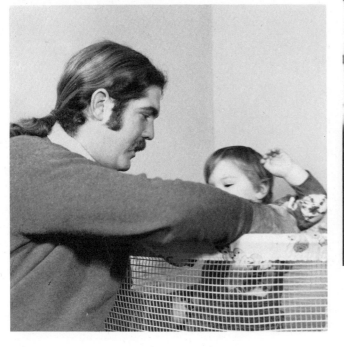

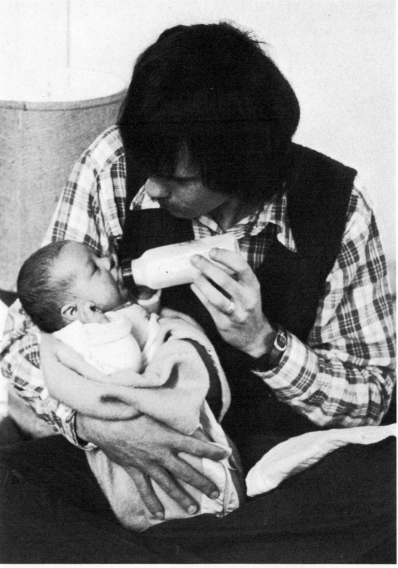

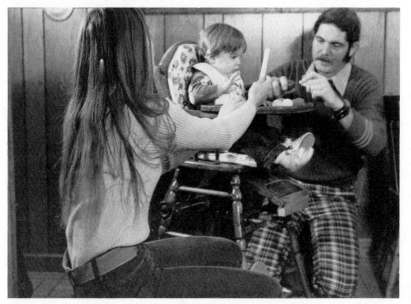

The only time I felt jealous—and it was more annoyed than jealous—was when the baby would start to cry when we wanted to go to bed together.

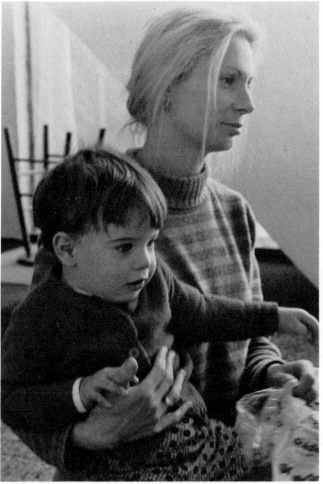

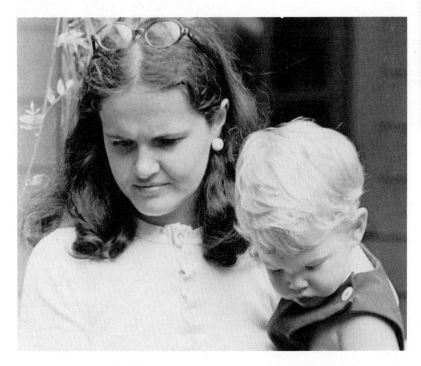

My husband's interest wasn't what I thought it should have been. He was in medical school and couldn't give lots of time or do lots of things. But I thought the baby was so fantastic. I was fascinated by everything he did. My husband didn't share that fascination. I don't know whether it worried me, or hurt me, or a little of both.

My husband saw our roles as structured. I thought it would be fine for him to change a diaper.

By the time the baby is six months old, most families are settling into their new state of being. The child is very much a person, responding to the parents and to the world around him.

Both man and woman are becoming increasingly identified with themselves as father and mother. The woman is making decisions about her life, is expanding her relationship to others and to the world outside as she comes out of the cocoon state when she and her child were totally interdependent. Both parents are beginning to deal with the baby as a personality, as someone who "talks" to them, calls to them to come, to wake up, laughs hysterically at a funny face or a tickling hand.

By now the woman should know and feel comfortable with her body, should be exercising it, using it, enjoying it. The mother and father now have some time for each other. The freedom of prechild days will never exist again. Even their grown child will be in their thoughts and a part of their concerns, but they now have their life together as well as their lives with their child.

The couple finds itself in a new social role; they are parents now. Somehow parenthood confers adulthood and recognition as a "real" member of society, as opposed to some free-floating being on the periphery.

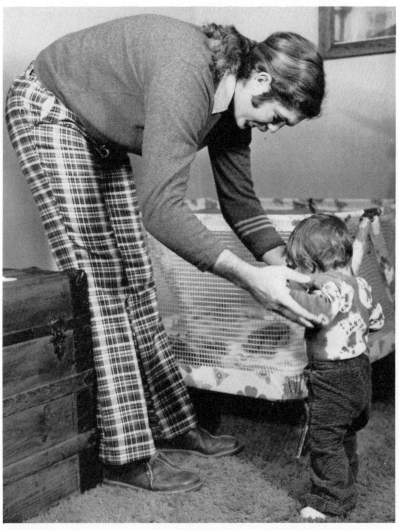

It's neat to come home to my wife and child. It makes it easier for me to go out and work, to do what I have to do.

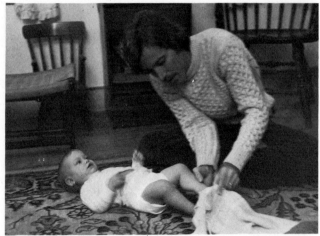

I wonder how she knows her father. She likes men, but she knows him!

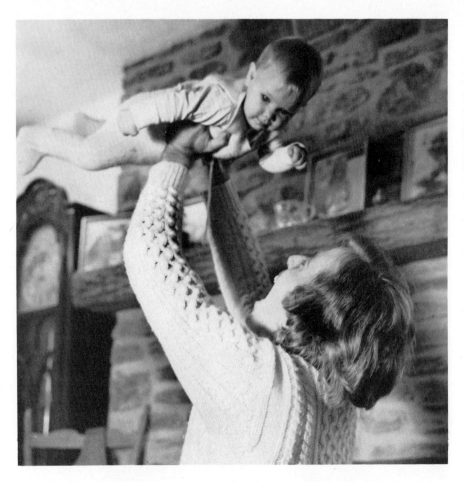

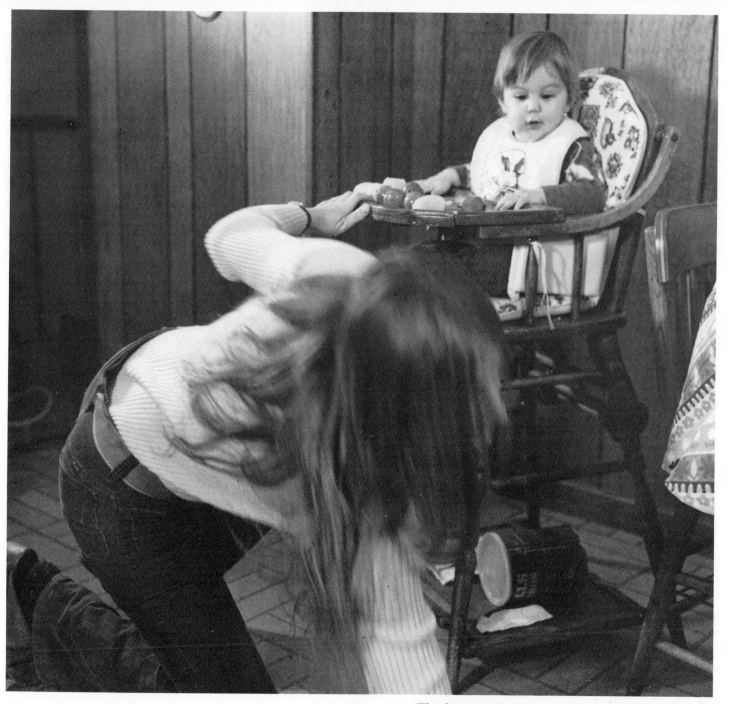

The days are a lot longer now; there's a lot more to do.

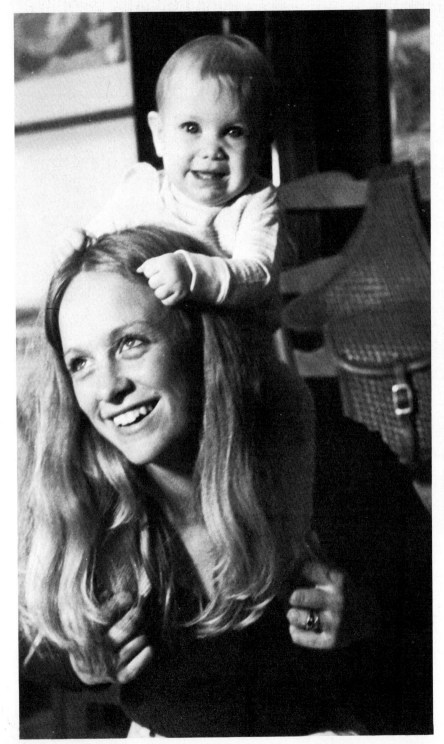

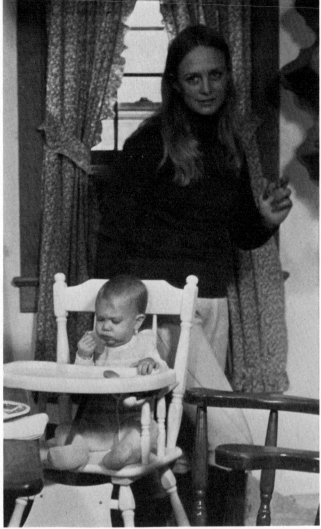

I've got the rest of my life to live with me. I have to satisfy myself, at the same time doing the best I can as a mother. If I deprived myself, I'd be a horrible mother.

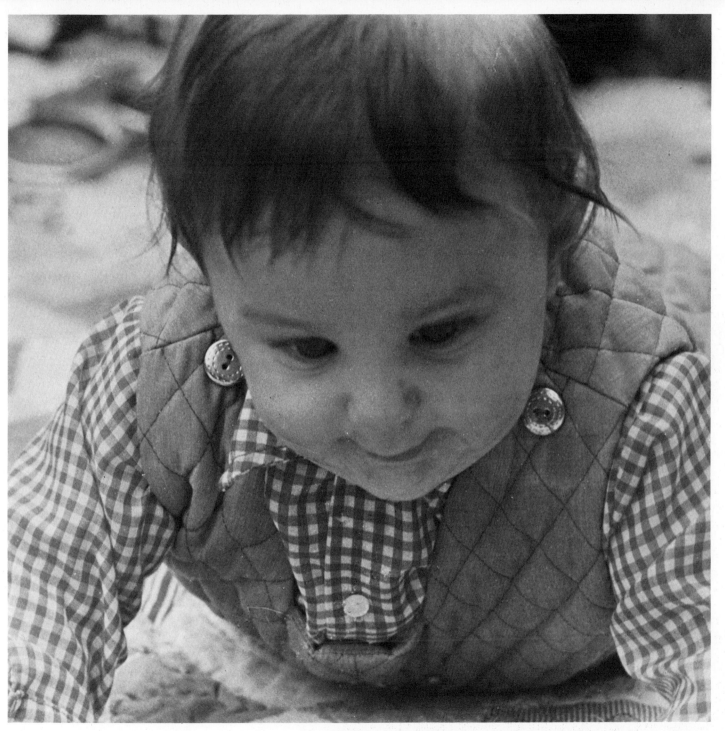

He rolled over today! Just one way though, from his stomach to his back.

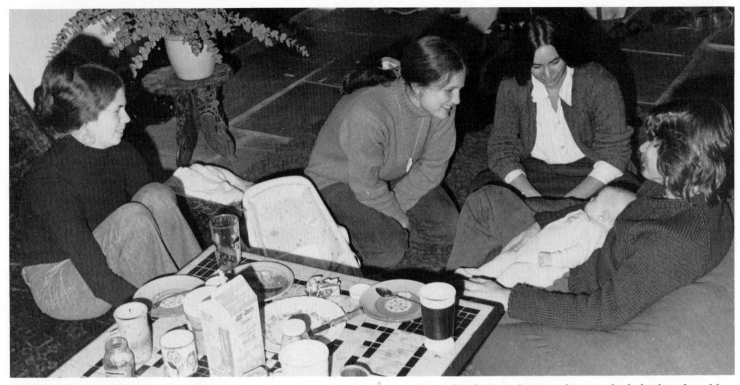

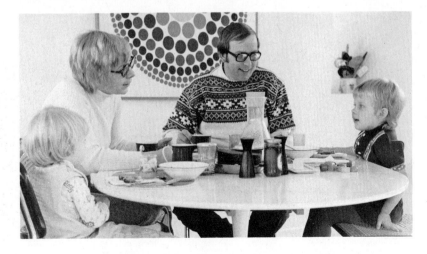

It used to be just the two of us—nobody bothered us. Now there are always people dropping in, or coming up to us in public places: "Oh, look at the baby!" "What a cute baby—may I hold him?" "Shouldn't you have him dressed more warmly?" And on and on. . . .

As soon as you have a baby, you're socially acceptable. Before that, you're out there somewhere. But once you're parents, you're accepted by people of any age: "Oh, they're parents now, it's all right."

I'm doing things I never thought I'd do, like having breakfast at seven in the morning, with my wife and children, before going off to work!

A child brings a sense of permanent attachment—a sense of family.

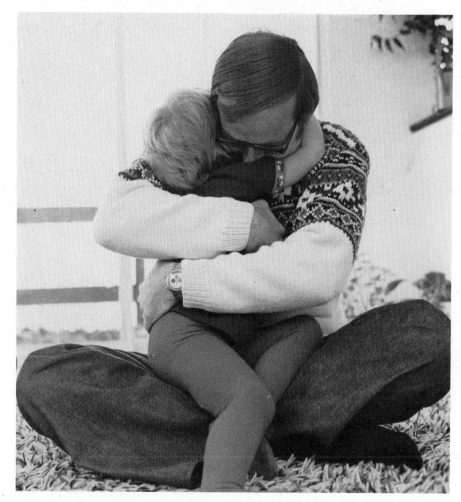

The Journey of a thousand miles
begins with one step.

—Lao Tzu

Parenthood is a never-ending journey, a never-ending learning experience, an awesome reminder of the passage of time as the children's birthdays slip by with ever accelerating speed. There is never a year of childhood as long as the first year of the first child. The focus on that child and the delights of seeing her traverse the evolutionary history of mankind are multifaceted and awesome.

By giving to our children, by accepting them as individuals, as separate human beings who have been entrusted to us for a short time while they become capable of functioning on their own, we can lose our ego involvement. Joy in parenthood and increased awareness of our own being comes when we can accept our children as they are, when we can give to them and expect nothing in return.

BIBLIOGRAPHY

PREGNANCY, BIRTH, AND PARENTHOOD

There are numerous books about babies, children, and parenting, many of them excellent. We cannot begin to list them all, so we have mentioned a few we think particularly good.

Arms, Suzanne and John. *A Season to Be Born*. New York: Harper Colophon Books, 1973.
A beautiful picture book, recounting the personal story of the Arms's pregnancy and the birth of their daughter.

Bing, Elisabeth. *Six Practical Lessons for an Easier Childbirth*. New York: Bantam Books, 1969.
The book giving the Psychoprophylactic (Lamaze) method of preparation for childbirth.

Brown, Buryn, Lesser, Mines, *Two Births*. New York: Random House/Bookworks, 1972.

Dodson, Fitzhugh. *How to Parent*. New York: Signet Books, 1970.
An excellent, all-round book with good sources, references, and bibliography.

Gattegno, Caleb. *The Universe of Babies*. Educational Solutions, Inc. 80 Fifth Ave., New York, N.Y. 10011.
Babyhood from the inside out.

Fraiberg, Selma. *The Magic Years*. New York: Charles Scribner's Sons, 1959.
Wonderful insight into the interior life of infants and young children.

Newton, Niles. *Family Book of Child Care*. New York: Harper & Row, 1957.
A complete book of child care by an outstanding author. Not nearly well enough known!

Rozdilsky, Mary Lou, and Banat, Barbara. *What Now? A Handbook for Parents* [especially women] *Postpartum*, 1972.
A wonderful booklet about all the nitty-gritty aspects of the postpartum period.

120

All of the above books, with the exception of *The Universe of Babies*, may be ordered from the ICEA Supplies Center, 1414 N.W. 85th Street, Seattle, Washington, 98117. They publish "Bookmarks," a book listing and review publication, and offer the most extensive list of pregnancy, birth and parenting publications available anywhere. Their mail order service is prompt and efficient.

YOGA

Be Here Now. Lama Foundation, Box 444, San Cristobal, New Mexico.
   A *beautiful* book!
Bhagavad Gita. Commentary by Swami Sivananda. The Divine Life Society, 1969. P.O. Sivanandanagar, Dt. Tehri-Garhwal, U.P., Himalayas, India.
   The Gita is the most important of all the Indian scriptures on yoga, as it is the culmination of all Indian thought to that date (200–500 B.C.).
How to Know God: Yoga Aphorisms of Patanjali. New York: Mentor Books, 1953.
   A modern retitling and translation of the *Yoga Aphorisms of Patanjali*, the only scriptural authority for the system of Raja Yoga.
Satchidananda. *Integral Hatha Yoga*. New York: Holt paperback, 1970.
   The most clear and concise book on Hatha Yoga available.
Suzuki, Shunryu. *Zen Mind, Beginner's Mind*. New York: Weatherhill, 1970.
   As close as words can get to describing the practice of meditation.
The Upanishads. New York: Mentor Books, 1957.
   Ancient writings on the nature of reality and spiritual consciousness.

INDEX TO HATHA YOGA POSES

AFTER THE BIRTH

BEGINNING AT HOME

WHEN YOU HAVE IT GOING

REGULAR PRACTICE

Don't forget Savasana between each of the poses

PHOTO CREDITS

ABOUT THE AUTHORS

Ferris B. Urbanowski served as instructor and adviser for *The Story of Eric*, and is the author of *The Lamaze Experience*, and *Practice for Childbirth*. Ms. Urbanowski has been an A.S.P.O. (American Society for Psychoprophylaxis in Obstetrics) certified instructor and parent educator since 1967. She is also an A.S.P.O. National Teacher Trainer and a student and instructor at the Center for Yogic Studies, Brookline, New Hampshire.

Balaram (William Francis Malloy), is the founder of the Center for Yogic Studies, New Hope, Pennsylvania and Brookline, New Hampshire, and was formerly with the Integral Yoga Institute, New York and Montreal. Balaram is a faculty member of Stroudsburg State Teachers College, Stroudsburg, Pennsylvania, and Bucks County Community College.